A History of
Mental Health Nursing

D1470694

B007232

The cover photographs convey strong impressions about mental nursing.

The picture of the gentleman on the tricycle was taken in 1892. He was a patient selected to be in charge of other patients working in the asylum gardens; because the gardens were so extensive, the superintendent provided him with a cycle. The phenomenon of patients supervising other patients happened frequently during the 19th and early 20th centuries.

The second photograph is of a group of female nurses and the superintendent. This picture is posed in a similar way to those taken of Florence Nightingale at St. Thomas's. The strong impression is created of a superintendent very much in charge surrounded by his female nurse attendants. These females were all qualified nurses. The picture supports the information given in the book that more females than males took the MPA examinations and passed them.

The last picture is an informal group of staff, patients and their relatives in the grounds of the Wiltshire Asylum in 1894. The informal pose suggests that there were times when staff and patients related to each other in a friendly and relaxed way. Both parties had a vested interest in ensuring that the asylums were well managed and ran at a profit.

A History of
Mental Health Nursing

Peter Nolan

Lecturer in Nursing Studies
University of Birmingham

CHAPMAN & HALL
London · Glasgow · New York · Tokyo · Melbourne · Madras

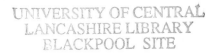
Published by Chapman & Hall, 2–6 Boundary Row, London SE1 8HN

Chapman & Hall, 2–6 Boundary Row, London SE1 8HN, UK

Blackie Academic & Professional, Wester Cleddens Road, Bishopbriggs, Glasgow G64 2NZ, UK

Chapman & Hall, 29 West 35th Street, New York NY10001, USA

Chapman & Hall Japan, Thomson Publishing Japan, Hirakawacho Nemoto Building, 6F, 1–7–11 Hirakawa-cho, Chiyoda-ku, Tokyo 102, Japan

Chapman & Hall Australia, Thomas Nelson Australia, 102 Dodds Street, South Melbourne, Victoria 3205, Australia

Chapman & Hall India, R. Seshadri, 32 Second Main Road, CIT East, Madras 600 035, India

Distributed in the USA and Canada by Singular Publishing Group Inc., 4284 41st Street, San Diego, California 92105

First edition 1993

© 1993 Chapman & Hall

This edition not for sale outside the USA and Canada

Phototypeset in 10/12 Times by Intype, London
Printed in Great Britain by T.J. Press (Padstow) Ltd, Padstow,

ISBN 0 412 39820 6
    1 56593 029 0

A catalogue record for this book is available from the British Library

Library of Congress Cataloging-in-Publication data available

For Mary, Sophie, Roisin and Alexandra

Contents

Acknowledgements

When I first began to work as a psychiatric nurse in the early 1960s, two observations forced themselves on me almost immediately. The first was the speed with which new ideas came into clinical practice, and the equal speed with which they became outdated and discredited; and the second was the capacity of psychiatric nurses to dwell on the past, on some golden age in nursing which had preceded the contemporary environment of change with which they had to contend. In their harking back to 'better' times, the nurses with whom I worked were undoubtedly no different from the general run of humanity with its tendency to glorify a past when they were not threatened by change. Nonetheless, it is to the nurses with whom I spent my initial years in psychiatry that I owe my first acknowledgement; they fed my interest in the development of psychiatric nursing, in its history and in nurses perceptions of their own past, an interest out of which, thirty years later, has grown this book.

I am also indebted to many other people for their help, guidance and support while I have been researching and writing this book. It would be impossible to mention them all by name. Retired nurses and others still embattled in the oft-times chaotic scenario of our present-day Health Services gave generously of their time in order to tell me their stories and give me their recollections of the past and opinions about the future. Their enthusiasm sustained me in my endeavours. There are some whose special help deserved my particular gratitude. They are Annie Altschul, John Green, Ronnie Newman, Olive Griffith, Michael Squizzoni, Pat Barry, Cliff Johnson, Christopher Maggs, Mike Smith, Ian Hollinsbee, and finally, Susan Floate and Margaret Harcourt Williams, librarians at the Royal College of Psychiatrists.

Introduction

The last 20 years have seen interest growing in both Europe and the USA in the history of psychiatry. This has come about largely as a result of the anti-psychiatry movement of the early 1960s which challenged psychiatry on many levels and forced a re-examination of its history, origins, claims and achievements. The leading figures in the movement – Laing, Szasz, Sedgwick and most notably, Foucault – were sceptical of the received wisdom amongst psychiatrists which was that the history of psychiatric care was predominantly their history, and this history one of straightforward and benign progress. As a result of the scepticism fed by Foucault, nurses have been empowered to ask why they have been allocated only a marginal role in the pages of history despite having had the most intimate therapeutic role in relation to the mentally ill. Why is so little known about the nurses of the past and their practices? In short, why has nursing been deprived of its founding fathers and mothers and left without historical role models, in a state of professional amnesia? One hundred years after the initiation of the first national training scheme for 'attendants upon the insane', it seems an opportune moment to take stock of where psychiatric nursing came from, and of how it developed, as well as looking at the major concerns which confront it as it approaches the millenium.

Having a history confirms the legitimacy of the service one provides: mere inclusion in the history of another group implies mere subordination. The history of psychiatry has taken many forms; there is the history of the institutions, of diagnosis and treatment, of particular practices, and of the lives of famous doctors (Marx, 1979). These histories have been written mainly by retired psychiatrists who have had particular messages to convey to a particular audience whose interest in nursing was minimal and satisfied by the most casual allusions to nurses. The majority of these historians have tended to see nursing as an integral part of psychiatry, with no separate existence from it. As is to be expected, the historian-psychiatrist's interest has been in the role and influence of medical people, and has tended to enhance these at the expense of the contribution made by other workers in the field of psychiatry. It may be that the reluctance felt by psychiatric nurses to examine their history is due to a feeling that what they will find there is not a portrait of themselves as they were, but a picture painted by a professional group which was basically disinterested in them.

However, the tendency of recent histories of psychiatry has been to point out that history is not solely about the great, the good and the powerful, but is also about the middle and lower ranks who have often been ignored. It is now widely recognized that the history of psychiatry is but one aspect of the history of mental health care. Walk (1961) declared that a history of psychiatry which did not include the history of mental nurses was incomplete. Hunter (1956) rejected the traditional historical image of the mental nurse as indolent, lacking in motivation, unable or unwilling to demonstrate compassion for patients, and so unintelligent as to be totally dependent on rules and routines. He argued that Britain led the world in reforming care of the insane along humanitarian lines. This care, he claimed, was directly related not to advances in drug therapy, or to sophisticated methods of restraint, but to the concern for suffering, the respect for individuals and the willingness to assist which characterized the nurses who cared for mental patients.

Digby (1985) found that asylum keepers and attendants were the 'hidden dimension' of the asylum system whose work has been rarely described. Russell (1983) also found that attendants were the backbone of the Victorian asylums, embodying the spirit of these institutions and exercising considerable influence over the lives of patients. Where doctors were anxiously striving to establish a knowledge base and rationale to support what they were doing, the work of the attendants was primarily with the patients, supervising them, exercising them, and frequently going beyond mere adherence to the Rule Book to provide comfort and support for them. Evidence is constantly accumulating which should empower nurses to disown the historical stereotypes with which they have been unfairly labelled. They can now begin to reconstruct their past without fear, and those entering the profession can be encouraged to participate in this enterprise and should benefit from it. It would be a mistake if students' timetables, already full of 'ologies' and 'isms' were to leave no space for reflection upon that very importance source of knowledge which lies in the past. It is also beneficial to disabuse students of the myth that everything contemporary is progressive and 'good' and everything that went before, primitive and 'bad'. The benefits of learning from history may be summed up by Santayana (1922), who remarked that those not conversant with the mistakes of the past are likely to repeat them in the future.

The purpose of this book is to examine mental nursing from a historical perspective, and to describe psychiatric nursing from the point of view of nurses. For the period prior to 1920, the book relies on written source material; but after 1920, the authentic voices of nurses who were working in the mental hospitals from the period between the First and Second World Wars until our own day can be heard through interviews carried out by the author. Nurses take centre stage in this account of the development of psychiatry and of care for mental patients, and the perspective thus afforded may, in some respects, be new and revelatory in comparison with other histories. The strategy of the book is to focus on certain periods in the history of mental nursing which are particularly enlightening in terms of demonstrating the challenges which have faced nursing through the years and the thinking which has met those challenges.

The book attempts to show how contemporary concerns in mental nursing have their origins in the past. The problems which bedevilled psychiatry in the early Victorian era have persisted through the decades and emerge, different only in the terminology used to describe them, in our own times. The aim of this book is to give mental nursing an identity of its own, separate from that of psychiatry, to win back for it its rightful place in the history of care of mental patients, and to empower it thereby to advance into the future with renewed vigour and confidence.

The book nonetheless deems it appropriate to spend time discussing psychiatry, both as a body of knowledge and as a practical discipline, because it is out of psychiatry that psychiatric nursing sprang. The annals of psychiatry reveal that it was doctors who employed nurses to work in the asylums; it was doctors who initiated the first training schemes for attendants; it was doctors who taught nurses during their training, who examined them, and who decided what the role of nurses should be. While the book aims to give an account of the history which has been too long neglected, it also recognizes that to offer a distillation of purely nursing experience would be to tell only a part of the story of caring for psychiatric patients. The history of nursing requires amplification from the histories of all the other groups who have worked in the field of mental health in order for it to be properly understood.

Nurses have struggled over the last 150 years to win recognition for the uniqueness of the contribution they make to patient welfare, and recognition that many elements of psychiatric care and treatment are delivered solely by them. Although the nursing profession today eagerly pursues the ideal that nurses should be autonomous practitioners, the history of mental health nursing does not reveal that nurses have ever been autonomous; they have always been closely linked to doctors and generally controlled by them. Over the years, nurses have changed the names by which they have called themselves but their attempts to separate themselves from medicine and the medical profession have largely been confined to these superficial changes in nomenclature. The history of nursing cannot be separated from that of the history of doctors in psychiatry.

Chapter 1 presents an overview of the book and discusses the different names by which mental nurses have been known over the last 150 years. The names are important in outlining, however simplistically, the way in which nurses perceptions of their role have changed during the last 150 years. Any book which attempts to cover two centuries of the history of psychiatry faces a problem of terminology in describing those who cared for the mentally ill. It would be anachronistic to refer to 'psychiatric nursing' in the context of the 19th century. This book, therefore, chooses to adopt the titles used to describe 'nurses' at the particular time under discussion. In later chapters, the book recognizes that the term 'patient' in the mental health context is now contentious and therefore prefers to refer to 'people with mental health problems'.

Chapter 1 proceeds with a discussion of the degree of kinship which nurses today have with the attendants of Victorian times. Major issues in mental nursing are identified and traced from the past into the present.

Chapter 2 looks at care of the mentally ill and examines the psychiatric literature pertaining to the period prior to the inauguration of formal training for the attendants in 1891. In Chapter 3, the beginnings of asylum nursing are discussed; the nature of the work of the attendants, their conditions of service and the kind of patients they cared for are outlined. The establishment in Britain of the first national training scheme for mental nurses is described in Chapter 4 and the consequences examined. Chapters 5 and 6 look at nursing in the early 20th century and onwards until the 1950s by studying the accounts provided by nurses who were working at that time. The influence of the anti-psychiatry movement is identified in Chapter 7 and the ideas of the great psychiatric reformers are contrasted with the practice of nursing as described by nurses who were working in the 1960s and 1970s. The 1980s are addressed in Chapter 8 – a decade of change in which the ideas of the 1960s were implemented in the closing down of the institutions and the advent of community-based care. Nurses then found themselves in search of a new role outside the hospitals, as they describe in their own words in this chapter. Finally, Chapter 9 reviews the themes which have persisted in nursing over the last 150 years and attempts to project into the future by considering issues likely to hold the attention of mental nurses as they move into the 21st century. The biggest issue of all is whether mental nursing can survive.

REFERENCES

Digby, A. (1985) *Madness, Morality and Medicine – A Study of the York Retreat*, Cambridge University Press, Cambridge.

Hunter, R. (1956) The rise and fall of mental nursing. *The Lancet*, **1**, 98–9.

Marx, O. M. (1970) What is the history of psychiatry? *American Journal of Orthopsychiatry*, **4**, 593–605.

Russell, R. (1983) Mental physicians and their patients. Unpublished PhD Thesis, Sheffield University.

Santayana, G. (1922) *Soliloquies in England and Later Soliloquies*, Constable, London.

Walk, A. (1961) The history of mental nursing. *Journal of Mental Science*, **107**, 1–17.

1

Psychiatric nursing: origins and contemporary issues

1.1 INTRODUCTION

This chapter gives an overview of the origins of psychiatric nursing and discusses some of the major issues which currently engage those involved in the training of nurses and in the management of nursing services. Since the establishment of the asylums and the advent of carers to work within them, nursing has always found itself sandwiched between those in pursuit of scientific certainty in the diagnosis and treatment of mental disorder, and those whose pragmatic approach to psychiatric institutions has seen them merely as centres for the dispensation of welfare. Thus hemmed in, nurses have rarely enjoyed access to the resources which would enable them to demonstrate fully the skills they have to ameliorate the worst conditions which can befall humanity. In the early days of the asylum system, their work was mainly confined to keeping the institutions clean and the inmates busy; during and between the First and Second World Wars, they were hampered by serious overcrowding in the asylums. In the late 20th century, it remains to be seen whether the community will be the context in which they can exert their skills to their maximum potential.

In its close alignment to the practice of psychiatry, nursing has suffered from the frequent therapeutic shifts which have taken place within that discipline over the decades. In its 19th century manifestation, psychiatry founded itself upon a medical model, attributing all mental illness to errors of biology; in the early 20th century, it was diverted from this model by practitioners in the newly emerging field of psychology who took it firstly in the direction of psychoanalysis and latterly, towards behaviourism. The medical influence reasserted itself in the middle part of the century when treatments such as electro-convulsive therapy, deep insulin therapy and chemotherapy became popular. In our own day, the most common approach to psychiatric illness used in hospital settings is the medical model, although many nurses working in the community find it unhelpful, preferring psychosocial models which favour the reskilling and empowering of patients to live their own lives (Cochrane, 1983; Simmons and Brooker, 1990). Thus caught up in the changing fashions of theory and practice, psychiatric nurses have experienced confusion about their own role, an uncertainty which has found itself reflected in the different names which nurses have favoured to describe themselves over the decades.

1.2 FROM 'KEEPER' TO 'MENTAL HEALTH NURSE'

The literature describing mental nursing in Britain towards the end of the last two decades of the 20th century employs four terms interchangeably: 'mental nurse', 'psychiatric nurse', 'nurse therapist' and 'mental health nurse'. The latter two reflect an unease with the term 'nurse' which some see as perpetuating the medicalization of those with a mental health problem and the supremacy of the medical model. The term most favoured in recent British nursing journals is 'psychiatric nurse' although, ironically, there is no such statutory qualification. The statutory training confers the qualification of Registered Mental Nurse (RMN) and the 1982 syllabus described itself as the Syllabus of Training for Mental Nurses. Project 2000 courses which were introduced in the late 1980s refer to the 'mental health nurse', a term which seems likely to take nursing into the 21st century.

During the 18th and early 19th centuries, the term 'keeper' was applied to those entrusted with the care of the mentally ill. 'Keeper' referred both to the owner of the house in which insane patients were cared for, and to those employed to run such houses. The term implied that those who looked after the mentally ill both restricted access to them and controlled the movements of patients in the same way that zoo-keepers and game-keepers controlled animals and game. With the emergence of the asylum system after 1845, the term 'attendant' was preferred as indicating a more humanitarian approach to care. The attendants 'attended' to the institution, keeping it clean and tidy, maintaining order by controlling inmates, and ensuring that there was sufficient farm and garden produce to render it viable. Attendants were also the medical superintendent's servants, with primary responsbility to carry out his orders.

From the mid–19th century, female attendants were generally referred to as 'nurses', although the men were still called attendants, but by the end of the century, 'nurse' had become a neutral term used for both male and female carers. In 1923, 'mental nurse' became the official title with the setting up of the Supplementary Register for Mental Nurses under the General Nursing Council (GNC). Nurses working at the Cassel Hospital in the early 1940s adopted the term 'psychiatric nurse', feeling that this change was justified because the treatment provided at the Cassel was based on a psychoanalytic model of mental illness, different from the treatment provided in traditional mental hosptials:

Nurses who worked at the Cassel in the early 1940s were specially selected, and indeed many were attracted to this new and exciting type of nursing.

Just as the type of work undertaken there was seen as being superior to what was taking place in other mental hospitals, so too the nurses saw themselves as being superior to other mental nurses. In assuming the title 'psychiatric nurse', they sought to indicate both their separateness and their superiority; but to other nurses the term 'psychiatric nurse' was a snobbish term. (Griffith, 1986, personal communication)

In the 1950s, American ideas and terminology were to the fore and doctors were influenced by what they read in the transatlantic journals. A junior doctor who spent some time in the USA after completing his training in Britain, was disturbed to note that American psychiatrists were basing their practice entirely on psychoanalysis, of which he had no understanding either from his own training or from what he had seen British practitioners doing. Although the young doctor found the kind of in-depth analysis which he observed strange in its intensity, a senior American doctor reproached him with the words:

This may seem funny to you, but to us, it is a religion. (Rollin, 1991)

The American writer, Hildegard Peplau, published her book *Interpersonal Relations in Nursing* in 1952 and this gave rise to the term 'psychodynamic nursing'. At the same time, nurses in this country were starting to hear themselves described as 'psychiatric nurses'. A nurse who worked in the Wiltshire County Asylum after the Second World War recounts how nurses who were doubly qualified in both general and mental nursing assumed the title 'psychiatric nurse'; they identified strongly with medical treatment of patients and considered it an important part of their role to assist with ECT, psychosurgery, deep insulin therapy and the administration of medications:

The rest of us were called 'mental nurses' or 'attendants', and we spent most of our time on routine duties, e.g. supervising patients in the airing-court, attending football and cricket matches, and accompanying patients to the weekly dances. In fact, we really got to know the patients, in some instances better than we knew our colleagues, and they in turn got to know us; you could say they saw us as friends. I have felt that the 'psychiatric nurses' regarded us as being inferior to them and not being as clever as they were; one thing is sure they spent as little time as possible with the patients. (Newman, 1986 personal communication)

Brooking (1985) suggests that nurses favour titles which reflect their own particular ideas about the nature of their work and of psychiatry. Some nurses see themselves as very much a part of a larger work-force in the field of mental health, a work-force which includes social workers, psychologists, occupational therapists and psychiatrists; these nurses would prefer a multidisciplinary approach to training and practice so as to break down the boundaries between professional groups and promote co-operation. At the opposite end of the debate are nurses who feel that they are first and foremost 'nurses' and only secondarily, nurses working with mentally ill patients. They feel that nursing has certain essential identifying features, irrespective of its area of practice: all patients have fundamental needs which must be met before any treatment can be effective. It is nurses who are the patients' advocates and the 24-hour-a-day service they provide differentiates them from all other health care workers.

1.3 INSTITUTIONAL PSYCHIATRY

The debate about the essential nature of nursing as reflected in the titles which nurses have adopted has continued for many decades. An examination of nursing history may help explain how there has come to be such a broad spectrum of ideas about the role of the nurse, and may also help nurses appreciate how such divisions have hindered nursing from progressing in a clear direction to the improvement of the status and effectiveness of the profession.

The 1890 Lunacy Act confirmed that the practice of psychiatry was firmly established within the walls of the mental institutions, those large, purpose-built edifices which were tactfully situated away from sane and sensitive Victorian society. Doctors had created for themselves a role and a sphere of considerable influence in the mental hospitals; psychiatry was becoming more and more 'respectable'. The position of those who nursed the patients was far less secure, less clearly defined and certainly less respected. The 'attendants' on the insane were just beginning, rather late in the day compared with asylum doctors, to organize themselves and to seek to have their role acknowledged and adequately rewarded. What exactly that role was was a perplexing question, remaining a cause for debate for many years, and still topical today as the care of those with mental health problems moves back into the community, taking, or perhaps not taking, psychiatric nurses with it. Late 20th century nurses are anxious about whether there is a place for them as health professionals to work with clients who have been discharged back into the community. Their dilemma is only an echo of Victorian nurses' efforts to convince others of the importance of the role of the trained psychiatric nurse within the mental institutions.

It is generally considered that modern psychiatry had its origins in the mid–19th century (Donnelly, 1983). Growing up alongside an expanding and flourishing industrial society was the belief that health could be made available to all through the interventions of science. The optimism that fired the magnates of the Victorian era equally fired society's conviction that many illnesses could be abolished, the severity of others ameliorated and some prevented altogether. Medicine and utopia went hand in hand. Not only were physical illnesses to be tackled and vanquished by science, but also those less tangible and more disturbing ailments of the mind.

A watershed in the care of the mentally ill was the 1845 Lunacy Act which compelled local authorities to make provision for psychiatric patients. Those who drew up the Act intended the concentrated and expensive public building programme which followed to represent the enlightened attitudes of their era, but it was certainly not without its critics. There were many who remarked that a building programme of such magnitude was squandering valuable resources on indolent and worthless individuals who most probably would not be able to repay society for the cost of housing them temporarily in an asylum. Sceptics asserted that the medical system which claimed to be able to treat and care for these patients was based on a set of untested assumptions. Equally dissatisfied were those who still felt that far too little was being done to help the weaker members of society. John Stuart Mill argued that the nation's moral strength lay not in how successful it was in imposing its rule on other people, but in how well it catered for its own poor, sick and enfeebled (Mill, 1978). The state expressed its humanity through its institutions.

The doctors who staked their claims to authority on the newly emerging scientific method willingly took on the task of identifying the mentally ill and those at risk of becoming so, of treating them and of returning them to the community, whole in mind and body, ready to play their part in the industrial and economic life of the country. Medical 'cure' and economic strategy thus went hand in hand; those who had been exposed to the therapeutic influence of the asylum would subsequently be able to contribute to the prosperity of the nation. Such was the growing stature of science, beginning indeed to replace or at least, redefine religious beliefs, that it seemed reasonable to assume that cures for mental illness would be as readily available as cures for physical ailments. Asylum doctors, trained in medicine and psychiatry (although training for both and particularly the latter was in its infancy) were entrusted with the management of the institutions and authority over their employees, including the nursing attendants.

There had been, in fact, little or no debate about the components of medical management or nursing care of the mentally ill. The asylum doctors hoped that answers to these questions would emerge in the course of their practice and observation of patients. The next 150 years suggested that their expectations were unfounded. The relationship between theory and practice, the former always lagging far behind rather than informing the latter, returned to haunt the providers of care again and again.

There was no lack of confidence, however, in the setting up of the asylum system. Indeed, the asylum buildings themselves were erected as if they were going to last forever. Their severe and awesome architecture had elements reminiscent of the aristocratic country house and the medieval monastery. The fine craftsmanship which was evident both on the facades and in the interior work represented civic confidence in the state, the organization of society and the power of scientific healing.

The history of care for the mentally ill since the 1845 Lunacy Act may be divided into four periods. The asylum period witnessed the establishment of an institutional base for the emerging discipline of psychiatry. This was a phase which crossed the Atlantic as a similar building programme was undertaken in America. The second period saw the demise of the term 'asylum' with a slight shift in public and medical thinking away from ostracizing asylum inmates, and the advent of the mental hospital. This shift was embodied in the Mental Treatment Act of 1930, a remarkably enlightened piece of legislation which defined the aims of psychiatry as treatment followed by rehabilitation, and which tried to eradicate the stigma of mental illness by introducing the era of the 'voluntary patient'. Psychiatric services, however, were still firmly located in the institutions. In the third period of the 1970s, some inpatient services were moved to District General Hospitals. This may have been another attempt to diminish the stigmatizing effects of psychiatric treatment by making it available in a neutral context and closer to the patients' relatives, or it may have represented psychiatry's attempt to consolidate itself within medicine and move closer to the centre of health service provision. The fourth and most recent period has seen the emergence of the community mental health team (CMHT) which seeks to provide a therapeutic and preventive service to people in a variety of settings, e.g. day hospitals, day centres, health centres, GP surgeries and in their own homes. This approach espouses the community care model in preference to the hospital system, and an individual approach to patients as opposed to a collective one.

The founding of the institutions and the evolution of psychiatry from collective control of large numbers of patients to an individual contract with each one have been the subjects of many studies. What has been very much neglected is the development of psychiatric nursing. The role that the attendants played during the formative years when the asylum system was becoming established, the role that nurses have played through the various changes in mental health care which have occurred since that time, and their role today and into the future still need investigation.

1.4 THE CREDIBILITY OF PSYCHIATRY

No analysis of the history and development of psychiatric nursing can be undertaken without first examining the evolution of psychiatry, because it was in the asylum culture created by psychiatrists that nursing emerged. Since the middle of the 19th century, the theory and practice of psychiatry have profoundly influenced nursing care. As psychiatry entrenched itself within the asylums, so the asylums became the domain of the attendants. Psychiatric nursing has, for the last 150 years had an institutional bias.

The early psychiatrists were neither scientists nor clinicians; their work was primarily custodial and experimental (Baruch and Treacher, 1978). They were guided by personal whims and pet theories about how asylums should be run and patients treated. It was in an attempt to gain vicarious respectability and establish a professional base within the asylums, that alienists (the term widely used for psychiatrists in the 18th and early 19th centuries) associated themselves with medicine (Ingleby, 1981). Some would argue that this leech-like adherence to medicine has been largely responsible for the failure of psychiatry to develop a coherent scientific identity of its own. It adopted the form of the medical model but there was little scientific content in its theories. This lack of a sound knowledge base has fuelled arguments still being strongly waged today about the origins and purpose of psychiatry.

There are those who would locate psychiatry within the positivistic scientific tradition which assumes that observations can be made objectively and that causal relationships which form the basis of the natural sciences can be applied to the social domain. The practice of psychiatry then becomes a scientific exercise, the foundations of which are grounded in the natural sciences (Mayer-Gross *et al.*, 1960). Positivism – the paradigm of studying human beings as if they were purely matter – has been frequently challenged:

> Treating people as if they were things is not only questionable methodologically, but it is a highly objectionable policy. This policy has to be understood as reflecting not the private attitudes of individual psychiatrists but the social role which psychiatry has acquired in the course of its history. The medical profession had no business dealing with mental problems because the problems were not usually physical in essence; doctors were no better equipped than the rest of us to understand human predicaments. Science only confused the issue because its fundamental premise, that people are like things and could be studied in the same way as things, was degrading and far fetched. (Baruch and Treacher, 1978)

Psychiatrists were 'bamboozled by their own scientific self-image', argues Ingelby (1981). They assumed a responsibility they could not meet and which was in excess of what society actually wanted them to do, which was to act as policemen of the insane. By describing patients as 'inadequate', 'morally defective' or 'abnormal', psychiatrists adversely influenced social attitudes already antagonistic towards the mentally ill.

The work of Clare (1982) is of particular importance when looking at the history of psychiatry and of nursing. He has provided a critical evaluation of psychiatry from the standpoint of the practising psychiatrist. He sees the problem confronting psychiatry as its lack of credibility both in the eyes of the general public and in the view of practitioners from other branches of medicine. As well as lacking a scientific identity, Clare notes that psychiatry has also suffered from poor leadership. Consequently, it:

> drifts from one meretricious explanatory theory to another, ready prey for

the competing ideologies that flourish in the wasteland which lies between the biological and the social sciences. (Clare, 1982, p. 21)

Coulter (1973), on the other hand, does not hanker after any explanatory theory, being convinced that the common sense on which psychiatrists rely in the absence of scientific back-up, is far superior to anything science could provide:

Psychiatric ascriptions are inescapably rooted in common-sense cultural understanding, and to imagine that they could be grounded in something which transcends common-sense, i.e. in neutral, scientific authority simply makes no sense. (Coulter, 1973)

The anti-psychiatrists of the early 1960s also renounced psychiatry's claims to scientific respectibility:

Much of what passes for medical ethics is a set of paternalistic rules, the net effect of which is the persistent infantilisation and domination of the patient by the doctors . . . Most people we call mentally ill impersonate the roles of helplessness, hopelessness, weakness and often bodily illness when, in fact, their actual roles pertain to frustrations, unhappiness and perplexities due to social, interpersonal and ethical conflicts. (Szasz, 1972)

Over a decade later, Szasz was even stronger in his repudiation of any scientific basis for psychiatry and, indeed, of its claims to be a branch of the medical profession at all. He saw it merely as fulfilling a role of social control:

I submit that the basic agenda of contemporary 'providers of mental health services' is the same as the agenda of madhouse keepers, alienists, and psychiatrists has always been – namely housing the homeless. (Szasz, 1985)

While not aligning himself with Szasz's wholesale condemnation of psychiatry, Clare (1982) asks practitioners to be aware of the limits of their knowledge and of the potential which the allied disciplines of sociology, psychology and anthropology have to inform and enrich the theory and practice of psychiatry. He is firm, however, in setting the limits of influence of these allied practitioners, warning them that they must operate within psychiatry 'with a sense of prudence and generosity'.

The call for 'prudence and generosity' reflects the fear of psychiatrists that the multidisciplinary approach is a potential threat to their power. Because Clare perceives limitations in non-medical approaches to mental illness which have not been subjected to 'rigorous scientific scrutiny', he invites psychiatry to dictate its own parameters and control infiltration by other disciplines. The options open to psychiatry are either to affirm its base in the biological sciences or to proceed in a direction hostile to medicine. With the second option comes 'holism' and what, in Clare's opinion, is the soft, doughy arena of gestalt psychology and encounter therapy which minister to the needs of people he sees as less ill than dissatisfied and more appropriately classified as demoralized than disordered:

> The further dilution of psychiatric theory by the woolier formulations of fringe psychotherapy would spell doom for psychiatry's efforts to establish for itself a sound foundation in the basic biological as well as the social sciences. (Clare, 1982, p.23)

Clare's argument seems to be that psychiatry should ground itself in the biological sciences, not because this will necessarily provide the best approach to understanding and treating the mentally ill, but because the alternatives are unproven. Professional appearance seems to have become confused with therapeutic success. Indeed, therapeutic success has largely evaded psychiatry whose patients relapse or require readmission on a scale unheard of in any other branch of medicine.

From the perspective of one in daily and intimate contact with physically and mentally handicapped clients, Vanier (1988) argues that to reduce care for vulnerable and powerless human beings to the level of models and theories is a grave mistake. Instead carers need rather to get close to people in their suffering by dropping their professional masks. True therapy lies in listening to clients' pain and developing levels of compassion and understanding that can convey to people that they are cared for.

1.5 CONFLICT IN PSYCHIATRIC NURSING

Nursing is perhaps the least isolated of professions and can only be studied within the far broader context of care and social organization. In their obsession with professionalization, for example, some nurse historians, argues Maggs (1984), appear to have overlooked the obvious fact that nursing is an economic activity. Nurses work and train in hospitals and institutions which were originally built at considerable expense and which remain in continuous interaction with local economies. The economic issue is one of many problems that psychiatric nursing is taking with it into the 21st century, problems which are certainly not new, although they may be couched in different terms. More than 150 years after the founding of the asylums, psychiatric nurses are still engaged in the quest for a unique role, a quest which often generates inter-professional rivalry, jealousy and suspicion.

Owens and Glennerster (1990) found conflict in all areas of nursing. In psychiatric nursing, the shift away from the hospitals to community care of the mentally ill, and the growing involvement of the independent sector have left nurses concerned and confused about their role in future mental health service provision. This confusion is made worse by the fact that the knowledge base of psychiatric nursing is still a contentious issue. Should training of psychiatric nurses be centred on the biological sciences or the social sciences, or should it focus on the acquisition of interpersonal skills? If a skills-based approach is adopted, will this result in the devaluation of intuition, compassion, personality and environment? Is there, in any case, sufficient understanding as yet of what skill is in relation to mental health care? What constitutes a skilful nurse? Until these questions are satisfactorily answered, is the pursuit of skills-based training realistic?

The demise of the Schools of Nursing, located within psychiatric hospitals, has wiped out one major source of recruitment into psychiatric nursing, and Project 2000 has gone further by reducing it to a branch programme. Some would see this as the death knell of psychiatric nursing and the first step in the direction of training a generic nurse (McIntegart, 1990). Others argue that the European influence in Britain could result not only in the elimination of the psychiatric nurse, but the erosion of psychiatric nursing skills (White, 1990). Those who see the situation more positively consider that nursing's newly forged links with higher education will strengthen its academic input, give nurses a sense of direction, and attract into psychiatric nursing people less dependent on traditional practices and more able to take the initiative. The advent of general management has significantly altered the career structure that was set up by the Salmon Report in the early 1960s for nurses who wanted to leave clinical practice and go into management. By the end of the 1980s, nurses were being encouraged to locate their careers within the clinical area.

The introduction of a mixed economy into health provision may, however, spell a very uncertain future for those engaged in caring for the mentally ill, an area not renowned for its attractiveness or its profitability. The prospect of assessing outcome by the number of patients processed leads to concern that psychiatric care may be measured in throughput rather than quality of care. Quality assurance models may focus on the environment of care and the sophistication of interventions at the expense of securing the quality of life of individual clients. In order to prevent this happening, consumer groups and those concerned with the welfare of psychiatric patients will have to direct their energies towards patient empowerment.

1.6 EMPOWERING MENTAL HEALTH CLIENTS

The work of Goffman (1961) persuasively argued against medical control of the mentally ill. It suggested that doctors had been largely unsuccessful in treating psychiatric patients during the 150 years in which they had dominated psychiatry. At one end of the spectrum of care, Goffman questioned the effectiveness of private psychotherapy purchased at great expense, and at the other end, of hospital care. His conclusions were that psychiatric hospitals had become dumping grounds for people whom society could find no better way of helping. Many patients, he claimed, improved in spite of hospitaliz-ation rather than because of it. In his view, hospitals stigmatize, alienate, and demoralize patients.

Professional neglect and the consequent suffering of mentally ill patients exposed by the public enquiries of the 1960s and 1970s awoke the campaign-ing zeal of the media. Television programmes and newspapers addressed the difficulties encountered by patients and ex-patients, and the charity MIND played a considerable part in putting the civil liberties of the mentally ill on the nation's social agenda. The response to overcrowding in the asylums and poor quality of care came in the 1980s with the switch to community care. Many felt that this shift would empower patients, turning them into health care consumers, clients within a market economy. Others argued that men-tally ill people had never had and would never have any power, and were not in a position to make choices in the market-place of services. Almost as soon as psychiatric patients had been placed in the community, there was criticism that most were leading empty lives on low incomes, in substandard accommodation. One commentator remarked acidly:

In the 19th century, mental patients were locked in and in the 20th century they are locked out. (Wallace, 1985)

If the shift to community care is to work effectively to the advantage of mentally ill clients, they must have access to housing which they can afford, and to regular employment; they need an income which is adequate to support a healthy and purposeful life-style. They need education to improve their skills and enhance their self-respect so that they can progress in indepen-dence. Above all, they need the support of professional staff who can encour-age, reassure and intervene if necessary. Levels of medication must be such as to facilitate quality of life rather than disabling the client.

Patient power has never been as well established in the UK as in the USA. The situation in Britain, however, is changing as the 21st century approaches. In the 1960s, psychiatric nurses were trained to manage wards; now their training emphasizes managing interpersonal relationships and assessing the patient's individual needs. The Griffiths Report (1983) recommended that the quality of health care should be measured by how it is perceived by clients. This denotes a radical shift from an era when the vested interests of professionals dictated what happened in patient care to a situation where the keynote is collaboration with clients. Collaboration with other providers of health services is also to the fore, and there is greater emphasis on health education, an area which has been significantly neglected by psychiatry in the past. The health care providers are to be made accountable to the recipients of care and to the community at large. Time will tell whether these aspirations are merely rhetoric or foundations upon which psychiatry can establish itself more firmly.

1.7 SELF-HELP AND SELF-HELP GROUPS

A noticeable feature of post-Thatcherite Britain in the 1990s is the increasing part in the health arena being played by self-help movements. These draw their strength from contemporary interest in issues surrounding consumer power, and aim to enable individuals to take responsibility for their own health. Groups of lay people who share certain life experiences come together to inform and support each other. Such groups have enormous potential for meeting members' needs and disseminating information to the public. The paradigm of people helping each other is much older than the paradigm of professional or specialist helpers providing services for a fee, this being a relatively modern development.

The increasing emphasis on the individual during the 1980s, both in the USA and the UK, resulted from government attacks on institutions such as the National Health Service (NHS) and education. At the height of her influence in Britain, Mrs Thatcher was propounding her belief that there is no such thing as society, but only individuals. The logical follow-on from such a view is to question whether the State should interfere at all in people's lives. The desirability as well as the viability of the welfare state was being questioned with consequent attacks on the NHS for fostering dependence, reducing people's motivation to look after themselves and decreasing choice, whilst encouraging spending, over-manning, specialization and bureaucracy. The idea of self-help appealed to politicians and others who wished to reduce state intervention and cut public spending.

The ethic of self-responsibility assumes that everyone has the ability to care for him- or herself, that everyone has equal access to health education, and sufficient income to lead a healthy life-style. It may not be realistic for vulnerable groups such as the poor, the poorly educated, the long-term unemployed, those with mental health problems, the elderly and the handicapped. Some would argue that a self-help ethos and self-help groups conceal gross deficiencies in social services, allowing government to side-step its responsibilities towards underprivileged sections in society. They may mask the real extent of serious social problems; it is noteworthy that with the discharge of mental patients into the community, there are now no accurate figures for the numbers of mentally ill coping by themselves, or for the numbers of homeless mentally ill or those attending GPs. Self-help may become a convenient way of making social problems disappear and to establish self-help services may be of greater priority to local authorities than the quality of the service and of the people delivering them (Ramon, 1991).

1.8 NURSES: ROLE AND ATTRIBUTES

Nurses, trained and untrained, form the largest group of those working within psychiatry, yet their history has received little attention. Impressions of attendants in the second half of the 19th century have to be drawn largely from the records of doctors and their *Journal of Mental Science*. The attendants appear to have been a largely uneducated, but very tractable labour-force, lowly paid and hard working, unable to secure more rewarding jobs elsewhere. By the 1920s, the work was still routine, unrewarding and low status, although many staff found hospital life tolerable because of its social, sporting and theatrical events. In the 1950s came the first studies to examine aspects of the nurses' work. The Liverpool Hospital Board study (*The Work of the Mental Nurse*) appeared in 1954; a similar study, of the same title, by the Manchester Hospital Board was published in 1956, and the works of Oppenheim and Ereman (1955), Maddox (1957) and John (1961) explored further the role of the mental nurse. The overall conclusion from these studies was that it was difficult to define psychiatric nursing because of its multiplicity of components.

In the late 1950s and 1960s, some studies examined the personalities and attitudes of nurses, and others tried to pin down the role of the psychiatric nurse. Rubenstein and Lasswell (1966) looked at how nurses were perceived by patients and concluded that:

The nurses were clearly regarded as part of the opposition . . . against whom the patient struggled to maintain his dignity, privacy and integrity. Nurses were always about at regular intervals during the night, awakening patients, nagging about getting dressed for breakfast, collecting laundry, serving meals, writing endless notes, handing out medications, enforcing rules and calling the doctor. (Rubenstein and Lasswell, 1966)

The same study found that qualified nurses did not challenge the rigid hospital hierarchy; they saw mental illness as a medical problem and bowed to the supremacy of doctors. In contrast, a study undertaken by the Ministry of Health in 1968 (DHSS, 1978) stated that psychiatric nurses were taking the initiative in providing counselling and psychotherapeutic services for patients, although, as Cormack (1975) remarked, there was no supporting evidence for this claim.

In the 1970s, Altschul (1972) studied the interpersonal relationships of nurses and patients and concluded that nurses mainly operated 'lay' or 'common-sense' perceptions of the mentally ill and that it was impossible to uncover any theoretical basis upon which they acted. Towell (1975) observed that psychiatric nurses undertook a variety of roles, but did not ascribe much importance to forming relationships with patients. In the same year, Cormack found that there was a wide discrepancy between the prescribed and actual roles of charge nurses.

This gulf between theory and practice was taken up in the 1980s by Powell (1982), who observed that what nurses were taught and the way in which they were taught did not help them in their day-to-day dealings with patients. The 1978 DHSS Report had noted that:

17

The greatest constraint placed on nurse training is the service role of the student nurses which has existed for more than a hundred years . . . older staff feel threatened by student nurses. (National Development Group, 1978)

With or without a service role, Brown and Walton (1984) considered that it is unwise to expect student nurses to change the system. Change cannot be brought about by classroom teaching alone and new basic training schemes. First, staff already in clinical practice have to receive intensive in-service education to help them understand and cope with change and to tell them what is expected of them in implementing it. Then the organizational climate of health care delivery must be addressed so that new thinking and practices can be accommodated, and this means that old-style paternalistic management structures must give way to management climates that facilitate change and improvement.

The 1982 Syllabus of Training for Mental Nurses aimed to change nursing practice in line with new ideas and to prepare nurses for work in the community. It claimed to give nurses a new direction and sense of professional identity, although much of the supposedly new knowledge contained in the Syllabus was already being incorporated into the practices of psychologists and social workers. This was the first Syllabus to be introduced without consultation with the Royal College of Psychiatrists and was thereby intended to signal that nursing was adopting a different and independent philosophical orientation from psychiatry. Training was no longer to be seen as a watered-down version of medical training; henceforth, caring for people was to be a different discipline from attempting to cure them.

The Syllabus was commissioned by the GNC 2 years before the Council was due to be disbanded. Arguably, the GNC had, in the past, accepted some of the responsibility for the low morale in psychiatric nursing. Its main concern had always been to amalgamate general and psychiatric nurses, and the latter group had been made to feel undervalued as a result. The haste with which the Syllabus was implemented was largely due to the observations and recommendations contained in the Jay Report (1979). The Report suggested that mental handicap nurses were inappropriately named and trained, their role being more educational than nursing. The Report recommended that they should be part of the social rather than the health services, and proposed that a single new profession be created for the care of people with a mental handicap. In order to prevent the same fate befalling psychiatric nurses, the GNC moved quickly to keep them within the boundaries of nursing. The speed with which the Syllabus was introduced prevented proper costing, nor were there any provisions made for its implementation. Most of its content was derived from humanistic psychology and 'talk therapies' which had their origins in the USA but which had not been evaluated in the UK.

For the first time, in contrast to previous syllabuses which had stressed what nurses should know, this syllabus spelled out what nurses should be doing. The skills defined in the Syllabus were derived hypothetico-deduct-ively from generalized concepts of what psychiatric nurses should do in the view of those entrusted with the design of the Syllabus. There was no evidence produced to indicate what patients found skilful in the behaviour of nurses.

In their critical analysis of the caring professions, Henley and Brown (1974) concluded that many of the 'skills' to which health professionals lay claim are merely ploys which enable them to make a living from the damaged psyches of others desperate for help. Their conclusion was that some 'trained helpers' are no more skilful than the man in the street, and 'some may be downright dangerous':

> The skills model is a liberal cover-up for power in therapy as in other professions. What therapists have is a monopoly not of knowledge, but of power. Even those therapists who feel themselves most powerless in their work-places must admit the contrast of their power with that of those whom they are to 'help'. And very often the power that the mental health professionals have is only that given them as servants of the more powerful; for preservation of the class structure is a very important use of the mental health establishment today. (Henley and Brown, 1974)

1.9 SUMMARY

The purpose of this book is not a critique of psychiatric nurse training nor a philosophical investigation into the nature of psychiatric nursing. Rather it aims to examine from an historical perspective how psychiatric nursing has arrived where it now stands at the end of the 20th century. The development of psychiatric nursing theory and practice may be interestingly and clearly traced through the changing patterns of nurse training since its inception for psychiatric nurses in 1891. And a second obvious, though often overlooked, source of challenging material relating to the historical and contemporary status of psychiatric nursing is in the accounts which nurses themselves, both old and young, trained many years ago and very recently, can provide. The book draws extensively on such first-hand accounts.

The proposition is that the problems surrounding the management of the mentally ill, the concerns of those who care for mentally ill clients, and the anxieties society has about both carers and patients are not new. Rather, they are problems which have beset psychiatry and psychiatric nursing from their inception. Until it is understood that only the language used to describe the problems has changed, progress into the future may be obstructed or impossible.

REFERENCES

Altschul, A. (1972) *Patient-Nurse Interaction: a study of interactive patterns in acute psychiatric wards*, Churchill Livingstone, Edinburgh.

Baruch, G. and Treacher, A. (1978) *Psychiatry Observed*, Routledge and Kegan Paul, London, p. 26.

Brooking, J. I. (1985) Advanced psychiatric nursing in Britain, *Journal of Advanced Nursing*, 10, 455–68.

Brown, J. and Walton, I. (1984) *How Nurses Learn: a national study of the training of nurses in mental handicap*, Department of Social Policy and Social Work, University of York.

Clare, A. (1982) Chapter 2, in *Psychiatrists on Psychiatry* (ed. M. Shepherd), Cambridge University Press, Cambridge.

Cochrane, R. (1983) *The Social Creation of Mental Illness*, Longman, London.

Cormack, D. (1975) A descriptive study of the work of the charge nurse in acute admission wards of psychiatric hospitals. Unpublished M. Phil Thesis, Dundee College of Technology.

Coulter, J. (1973) *Approaches to Insanity*, Martin Robertson, London, p. 32.

Department of Health and Social Security (1968) *Psychiatric Nursing: today and tomorrow*, HMSO, London.

Donnelly, M. (1983) *Managing the Mind*, Tavistock, London.

Goffman, E. (1961) *Asylums*, Penguin, Harmondsworth.

Griffiths Report (1983), *Recommendations on the Effective use of Manpower and Related Resources*, HMSO, London.

Henley, N. and Brown, P. (1974) The myth of skill and the class nature of professionalism, in *The Radical Therapist*, Radical Therapist/Rough Times Collective, p. 62. Penguin, Harmondsworth.

Ingleby, D. (1981) *Critical Psychiatry: the politics of mental health*, Penguin, Harmondsworth.

John A. (1961) *A Study of the Psychiatric Nurse*, Livingstone, Edinburgh.

Maddox, H. (1957) The work of mental nurses. *Nursing Mirror*, p. 105.

Maggs, C. (1984) A new history of nursing – changing perspectives. *Nursing Times*, 80, 19–25.

Mayer-Gross, W. Slater, E. and Roth, M. (1960) *Clinical Psychiatry*, Cassell, London.

McIntegart, J. (1990) A dying breed. *Nursing Times*, 86, 72.

Mill, J. S. (1978) *On Liberty*, Penguin, Harmondsworth.

National Development Group (1978) *Helping Mentally Handicapped People*, Department of Health and Social Security, London, p. 78.

Oppenheim, A. M. and Ereman, B. (1955) *The Function and Training of Mental Nurses*, Chapman & Hall, London.

Owens, P. and Glennerster, H. (1990) *Nursing in Conflict*, Macmillan, London.

Peplau, H. (1952) *Interpersonal Relations in Nursing*, G. P. Putman's, New York.

Powell, D. (1982) *Learning to Relate*, RCN Publication, London.

Rollin, H. (1991) Address to the Royal College of Psychiatrists Annual Meeting: 150 Years of Psychiatry 1841–1991. Brighton.

Rubenstein, R. and Lasswell, H. (1966) *The Sharing of Power in a Psychiatric Hospital*, Yale University Press, New Haven, p. 55.

Simmons, S. and Brooker, C. (1990) *Community Psychiatric Nursing: a social perspective*, Butterworth-Heinemann, London.

Szasz, T. (1972) *The Myth of Mental Illness*, Harper and Row, London, p. 26.

Szasz, T. (1985) *Towards a Whole Society*, Richmond Fellowship Press, London, p. 40.

Towell, D. (1975) *Understanding Psychiatric Nursing*, RCN Publication, London.

Vanier, J. (1989) Foreword, in *Sharing the Darkness* (ed. S. Cassidy), Darton, Longman and Todd, London.

Wallace, M. (1985) When freedom is a life sentence, *The Times*, 16 December.

White, E. (1990) *The Future of Psychiatric Nursing by the Year 2000: a Delphi study*, Department of Nursing, University of Manchester.

In search of the roots of psychiatric nursing

2.1 INTRODUCTION

Professional groups may find it in their own interests to claim a long and exalted history of service to the community. Such a history may enhance their status and thereby increase their power and income! It may be the case, however, that a profession associates itself with certain activities which took place in the past but which, on closer analysis, turn out to have no direct link with the activities which that profession is engaged in today. Whether those who now care for the mentally ill have anything in common either as individuals or in terms of the work they are doing with those who were associated with the mentally ill in previous decades is subject for legitimate enquiry.

A review of the literature surrounding the history of British nursing suggests that, at best, psychiatric nursing has been considered an appendage either of general nursing or of medicine and, at worst, an irrelevance meriting little or no acknowledgement in the history of care. This is a lamentable omission because care of the mentally ill has a long and rich tradition and to tell its story should be of great significance to psychiatric nurses. As has been argued:

> Lack of appreciation of the past tends to foster over-evaluation of modern achievements and the assumption, so stultifying to progress, that what is present is good and what is past is bad. (Hunter and Macalpine, 1970, p.3)

Societies have always sought to identify and contain madness. In Britain, as elsewhere, many ways of warding off, categorizing and curing madness have been tried. Responses to madness have varied with changes in religious beliefs, and with shifting intellectual currents. Political and social prejudices and fears have played their familiar parts (Clarke, 1975).

The treatment of mental disorder can be traced back to antiquity (Hunter and Macalpine, 1974). The Greeks had a well-established system of care. To elicit the state of mind of the mentally disturbed person, Cicero designed an interview format which contained the following items (Clarke, 1975, p. 21).

1.	Nomen	Clan/tribe, region, connections
2.	Natura	Sex, nationality, family status, age, physique
3.	Victus	Education, association, habits/life-style
4.	Fortuna	Rich/poor, free/slave, social class
5.	Habitus	Appearance
6.	Affectio	Passions, emotions, temperament
7.	Studium	Interests
8.	Consilium	Motivation
9.	Factum	Working history
10.	Casus	Significant life events
11.	Orationes	Form and content of discourse

This assessment tool was used throughout the Roman Empire. Seranus, a Roman physician and teacher, was an advocate for a compassionate and civilized approach to the insane. He considered that sufferers needed to be understood, and, as far as possible, to be protected from fear, anger and blame. They should be exposed only to the companionship of non-threatening persons who could engage them in discourse, join them in reading and share the delights of music and the enjoyment of long walks. For Seranus, healing was contingent upon the caring relationship.

In discussing mental disorder in early Britain, Clarke (1975) examines the Celtic Church's organization and delivery of care. Attached to each monastery were a number of itinerant monks known as 'soul friends' who made mental health their particular concern. It may perhaps be stretching the imagination too far to see these as the forerunners of community psychiatric nurses! Their role was to befriend the disenchanted and melancholic and to form intimate spiritual relationships with the afflicted so as to 'steer them back' into social harmony with kith and kin. Some island monasteries allowed 'penitents', or those who were profoundly disturbed, to live with the monks and participate in their daily work and spiritual exercises. A monk from the 9th century, named Guthlac, offers one of the earliest written diagnoses of a depressive disorder:

> The ancient enemy of the human race shot the poisoned arrow of despair right into the centre of his mind. (Clarke, 1975, p. 50)

According to manuscripts belonging to the Celtic monasteries, Cicero's interview format was widely used by the monks. It may have been brought over by physicians who accompanied the Romans when they occupied Britain. Clarke finds that it was still in use at the time of the Dissolution of the Monasteries, but subsequently fell into abeyance.

Shrines were places of healing in both pagan and Christian times. Foucault

(1965) has remarked that many present-day mental hospitals are built on or near the sites of former shrines. The most famous shrine in Europe was probably that of St Dymphna in Belgium where the therapeutic community of Gheel grew up from the 13th century. There the mentally disordered were provided and cared for until they were sufficiently well to contribute to the upkeep of the community (Jones, 1983). Shrines were often associated with springs and wells. Such was their reverence for fresh water that our ancestors regarded the places in which it could be found as sacred. The sick of medieval times often travelled long distances to such freshwater sources and were accompanied by carers who 'guided' or 'attended' them. Healing, it was thought, could only take place if both guide and sufferer shared an unquestioning faith that recovery was possible. Failure to get well was therefore attributed to one or other's lack of conviction.

Water has always held a fascination for healers. From ancient times, its cleansing action was made much of by those who held the view that illness, mental and physical, was the result of sin, uncleanliness or impurity.

> Water could be used either actually or symbolically to wash away the offence. Thus, washing and purification were an essential preliminary to the healing process. An inscription over the entrance to the temple at Epidauras reads: 'Pure must he be who enters the fragrant temple; purity means to think nothing but holy thoughts'. (Jones, 1983, p.5)

Churches and hospitals were built where there was a ready supply of fresh water. Mineral water was used to purge patients and thereby promote inner cleanliness. More recently, in the 18th century, the spa towns enjoyed economic prosperity and the favour of high society because of the supposedly medicinal properties of their waters; in the middle to late 19th century, the working classes expressed their sense of the healing properties of water by making popular the seaside resorts.

In medieval England and Europe, the Church was an important provider of care for the poor and the insane:

> In medieval times, the duty of relieving the poor, though legally incumbent upon the Manor (the Landowner) was generally recognized as morally falling upon the Church. (Tate, 1969)

The Church wielded considerable power, not only as the dispenser of welfare, but also in influencing social attitudes. Two notables who came under the influence of the Church were St John of God and St Vincent de Paul, who devoted themselves to the service of the insane. Jaco Cuidad (1495–1550) was born in Portugal and spent most of his life travelling and working as a shepherd, soldier, labourer and bookseller, until he finally settled in Granada. There he underwent a conversion experience so dramatic in its intensity that he was placed in a hospital for the insane – the equivalent of a life sentence! There he was subjected to gross humiliations and severe beatings. Due to the efforts of an influential friend, he was finally discharged from the hospital having gained a profound insight into the care and needs of the sick and insane. Thereafter, he founded a house in Granada where mentally ill people and other social outcasts could come for care. His followers formed the Order of the Brothers of Charity and Jaco Cuidad was canonized as St John of God in 1690. The Order spread throughout Europe, being particularly strong in France, Poland and Bohemia. Today, nearly 2000 'Hospitallers', as members of the Order are called, administer some 200 hospitals, in addition to clinics, homes for the physically and mentally handicapped, and for alcoholics and geriatrics, throughout the world (Purcell, 1982).

St Vincent de Paul (1580–1660) undertook similar work to that of St John of God, redirecting the leper hospital of St Lazarus in Paris to the care of the mentally ill. He assisted Louise Marillac in founding the Order of the Sisters of Charity whose work included caring for female mental patients. Both these humanitarian figures were powerful in attracting others to the service of the poor and rejected.

2.2. CARE OF THE MENTALLY ILL IN THE 17TH TO 19TH CENTURIES

We are accustomed to thinking of the 17th century as a time of tremendous energy in the arts, in politics, in science and in philosophy. Such dynamism was evident also in the writings of contemporary physicians. The study of Edward Jorden (1569–1632) on hysteria rejected medical treatment for this condition, considering that a kindly carer had far more to offer. Jorden found that there were three elements of care: firstly, the carer should be in empathy with the distressed person; secondly, care should be offered within an understanding community; and thirdly, prior to any medical interventions taking place, the sufferer's fully informed consent should be sought. This would enable carers to establish relationships with clients based on honesty and trust (Hunter and Macalpine, 1970).

Writing from personal experience, an excellent commentary on psychiatric care was provided by James Clarkesse in 1679. He had been a clerk in Samuel Pepys' office before falling sick and being admitted to a private madhouse in Finsbury. His description of his experiences there was written in verse. He addressed the keepers, reminding them that violence against patients would produce violent patients and that:

> Porters and Keepers when they're civil,
> They charm in me the madmen's Devil,
> The Roaring Lion turns to Lamb,
> Lies down and couches wondrous tame.
> (Hunter and Macalpine, 1970, p.215)

The non-conformist minister, Timothy Rogers (1658–1728), wrote detailed instructions in his *Advice to Friends of Melancholy People* on how to care for patients suffering from 'trouble of mind':

1. Look upon your distressed friends as under one of the worst distempers to which this miserable life is obnoxious. Melancholy seizes on the Brain and Spirits, and incapacitates them for thought and action: it confounds and disturbs all their thoughts and unavoidably fills them with anguish and vexation.
2. Look upon those that are under this woeful disease with great pity and compassion. Do not use harsh speeches to your friends when they are under this disease.
3. Do not much wonder at anything they say or do. What will not people do that are in Despair! What will they not say that think themselves lost forever!
4. Do not think it altogether needless to talk with them. It is the length of their trouble that amazes them, when after one week, or a month, without sleep or rest or hope, and still the next week or month is as painful and as terrible to them as the former was. (Hunter and Macalpine, 1970, p. 248–51)

William Battie (1703–1776) was a pioneer in the care of mental patients. As a physician of high repute with a scientific background and distinguished social position, he helped raise the 'mad business' to a respectable medical speciality. It is rather unfair to his humanitarian zeal that the popular derogatory term 'going batty' should have been derived from his name! William Battie was the first public figure to recognize that mental nurses needed to be specially selected and carefully trained. His call for a better class of person to become 'attendants to the mentally disordered' was to be repeated frequently in the later history of mental nursing. Battie noted that some patients recovered without treatment, or only after treatment had been stopped, and this observation led him to consider the powerful therapeutic effects of a caring environment.

John Strype (1642–1737), an ecclesiastical historian and antiquary, writes about Bethlem Hospital at the end of the 17th century. The staff included 'three Basket Men' – the predecessors of psychiatric nurses – whose title derived from the days when Bethlem was a monastic foundation and monks with baskets went out to collect food and alms for the sick. Inside the front door of the hospital was hung a set of rules headed 'An Abstract of Orders of Court made on the 30th March 1677 for the Good Government of the Hospital'. The Orders stated:

That the bell be rung at sunset every evening, summer and winter, and that persons do depart.

That no person do give the lunatics strong drink, wine, tobacco or spirits, nor be permitted to sell any such thing in the hospital.

That such of the lunatics as are fit be permitted to walk in the yard till dinner time, and then be locked up in their cells and that no lunatic that lies naked or is in the course of Physic be seen by anybody without order of the physician.

That no servant whatsoever shall take any money given to the lunatics, to convert the same to their own use, but the same to be kept for the lunatics till recovered, or laid out for them in the meantime as the Committee thinks fit.

That no Officer or Servant shall beat any lunatic, nor offer any force to them, but upon absolute necessity for the better governing of them.

That some of the Committee go weekly to the said hospital to see the provisions weighed: and that the same be good and rightly expended. (Hunter and Macalpine, 1970, p. 309)

Strype visited the Bethlem Hospital frequently and considered the conditions there very good. He wrote that no patient had ever been recorded as running away, and that two out of every three were discharged, apparently 'cured', after an average stay of only 2 months.

The Committee Books of Bethlem from the 1760s and 1770s show, however, that the Basket Men were frequently reprimanded for negligence. It was written on 19 October 1771, that the cost of recapturing an escaped patient would be deducted from the pay of the person deemed to be responsible for having allowed the escape to occur. Further notes indicate that the 'servants' frequently had to be reminded of the importance of their role and of the high standards they were expected to maintain.

The picture which the Committee Books paint of the work of the Basket Men reveals the still lingering influence of medieval monasticism on the running of the Hospital. There was a strong emphasis on order and rule-keeping and the ringing of bells. The fact that the Orders of Court were inscribed on the wall of the Hospital was a constant reminder to the staff that they were under surveillance and would be punished if they transgressed. The staff acted as instruments of the governing regime. Because they were in general poorly motivated and untrustworthy, they were closely controlled and independence of clinical practice was unthinkable. Nonetheless, their role was seen as vital.

The physician, Thomas Withers, (1750–1809) considered that the key function of the keeper was:

Not to allow patients' minds to remain idle, but to keep them occupied with work which they prefer, filling their time with entertainment and amusements. (Hunter and Macalpine, 1970, p.464)

27

He highlighted the importance of 'companionship' between patient and keeper. The right kind of staff could engage patients in conversation and motivate them to useful work.

Dr Nathaniel Cotton, who ran a private madhouse at St Albans, attached the highest importance to the 'servants' he employed. His establishment enjoyed a good reputation, and one of his clients was the poet, William Cowper, who observed of the physician that he was 'a man well known for his humanity and sweetness of temper'. Cowper spent nearly 18 months from 1764 to 1765 at St Albans and during that time, Dr Cotton visited him every morning and 'delightful themes from the Bible formed the basis of our conversation'. Besides Dr Cotton himself, the home was evidently blessed with excellent attendants; of his own attendant, Sam Roberts, Cowper wrote:

> He maintained such an affectionate watchfulness over me during my whole illness, and waited on me with so much patience and gentleness, that I could not bear to leave him behind, though it was with some difficulty that the Doctor was prevailed on to part with him. (Cowper, 1816)

Shortly after the poet left St Albans, the attendant joined him in his new house in Huntingdon near Cambridge. Cowper felt that his nurse protected him from the harshness of the world by looking after him with a father's protective and tender care. Although he suffered from depression until the end of his life, the poet never again had to enter a madhouse, a circumstance which he attributed to the services of his attendant.

Some private madhouses extended their psychiatric services to the support of clients in the community. Dr Hill ran an institution for the 'medical treatment and care of persons afflicted with mental disorder' which adjoined his own residence in Leicester. He advertised his facilities in local papers and stated that experienced attendants, male or female, would be sent any distance to convey patients to his institution. Attendants could also be provided to live with and look after patients in their own homes or in lodging houses (*Aris's Gazette*, Birmingham, 12 January 1818). Such attendants were in many respects forerunners of modern community psychiatric nurses.

In France, thinking about the role of the attendants was developing along similar lines to those being explored in England. M. Berthier, physician of the Asylum of Bourg, considered that the essential qualities of attendants were health, morality, intelligence and charity; he also required a sense of duty, obedience, order and cleanliness. Sadly, he was forced to recognize that candidates of such stature were not forthcoming, and turned instead to members of religious orders whom he thought could be employed in asylums as long as they were prepared to submit to the will of the Physician Superintendent! (*Journal of Mental Science*, Vol. 9, 1863).

One of the great French psychiatric reformers, Pinel (1745–1826), bore witness to the skills and vision of the Head Attendant at the Bicetre Hospital, Jean-Baptiste Pussin. Pussin and his wife had initiated humanitarian reforms before Pinel was appointed there and then supported the doctor in implementing new schemes. Pussin, stated Pinel, exercised 'the vigilance of a tried and watchful parent . . . and cruel treatment of every description was banned' (Walk, 1961). Pussin had himself been a patient at the Bicetre, suffering, it is believed, from depression in his early years, and it became policy there to choose staff from among recovered or convalescing patients. This practice was enthusiastically approved of by Pinel, who described these recruits as best placed to understand the needs of the inmates as a result of what they themselves had experienced. Husband and wife teams were a feature of asylum organization in the early 19th century, many sharing their home life with the patients in their care. Jones (1983) refers to Catherine Allen who married George Jepson, Head Attendant at the Retreat, and became the first Matron there:

> Mrs Jepson's tea parties had a valuable socialising influence on the patients. (p. 126)

Catherine had gained her early experience of caring for mentally ill patients at Brislington House, a private Quaker establishment near Bristol run by Dr Edward Fox. Her compassion and dedication won the admiration and gratitude of her patients and their families. With her husband at the Retreat, she ran a humane and efficient organization until their retirement in 1823.

Another such couple were Dr and Mrs William Ellis who were appointed to the Hanwell Asylum in 1831. Mrs Ellis acted as Matron and took upon herself the role of the present-day occupational therapist, while her husband agitated for better pay for 'keepers' so that more 'respectable' persons might be attracted to the work. Dr Ellis also wanted attendants to receive training so that they might legitimately be referred to as 'nurses'. In his book, *Treatise on Insanity*, published in 1836, he uses numerous examples of how good nursing practice can calm agitated patients, encourage the depressed and give hope to the hopeless.

2.3 POVERTY, INSANITY AND THE WORKHOUSES

The patients who came under the humanitarian regimes of Jepson and Allen or of the Ellises were the lucky ones; most fared far worse at a time when there was much fear of mental illness and lack of understanding of the needs of mental patients. Provision varied greatly throughout the country; there was no uniform system of care. Private madhouses might take just two or three 'patients' or several hundred. They were run primarily for profit and the majority provided merely the basic necessities of life. Only a few engaged the part-time services of a physician and the number of staff was kept to a minimum. Conditions were generally such as to promote mental disorder rather than cure it. The owners of private madhouses were paid an allowance for each inmate by the parish and their obligation was only to control and supervise the 'patients'.

Dr John Haslam writes about the keepers at the London asylums in the early 1800s in his book *Observations on Madness and Melancholy*, published in 1809. He found that the quality of care in the public asylums was superior to that in the private sector:

> With respect to the persons, called keepers, who are placed over the insane, public hospitals have generally very much advantage. They are better paid, which makes them anxious to preserve their situations by attention and good behaviour: and thus they acquire some experience of diseases. But it is very different in the private receptacles for maniacs. They there procure them at a cheap rate: they are taken from the plough, the loom, or the stable; and sometimes this tribe consists of decayed smugglers, broken excise-men, or discharged sheriff's officers. If anything could add to the calamity of mental derangement, it would be the mode which is generally adopted for its cure. Although an office of some importance and great responsibility, it is held as a degrading and odious employment, and seldom accepted but by idle and disorderly persons. (Haslam, 1809)

The only way to control such a work-force was to devise rules for every moment of the day and for every eventuality, and then to enforce the rules rigorously. Duddeston Hall, an early 19th century private asylum in Birmingham, displayed its rules in its front entrance, rules which related to all aspects of asylum life:

> Every keeper and servant is expected to rise at 6.00 a.m. The keepers, after washing and combing the patients, will then proceed to examine them for injuries, rashes or sores. After this, the staff are expected to examine the stools and urine of the patients so as to be able to report the state of the patients.

Scull considers that the position of the 'insane class' in Britain between the medieval period and the beginning of the Industrial Revolution was far superior to their circumstances in later decades. In the middle ages, the mad had at least been left to their own devices:

> The deranged beggar was a familiar part of the medieval landscape, wandering from place to place in search of alms. (Scull, 1982)

By the middle of the 18th century, the insane were increasingly being brought under a surveillance often singularly lacking in compassion. if they were unable to work, the Poor Law confined them as pauper lunatics in workhouses under the supervision of a parish overseer. Those who fell foul of the law were detained in houses of correction (bridewells) and the Vagrancy Law dealt similarly with those who wandered beyond the confines of their parish. In the absence of public asylums, confinement meant:

> Either the ordinary poor-house or else, if they seemed dangerous, some disused building or some den where they could be put away in safety. (Henriques, 1979)

Workhouses had been established in the 1630s to cater for the poor among whose number were many insane. From 1760 onwards, more workhouses were built as these institutions tended to become dumping grounds for the dependent of all description (Henriques, 1979). The workhouses were managed on the philosophy that their inmates were poor because they were idle and therefore in need of reform. Hard work of a penitential nature was considered appropriate: beating hemp, dressing flax, carding and spinning wool, stripping and rolling tobacco and picking oakum.

The long French Wars at the end of the 18th century impoverished the nation and a series of catastrophic harvests inflated the price of bread above what the poor could afford. The industrialization of the early and mid–19th century served only to deepen the gulf between the rich and the poor rather than bringing affluence to the whole nation. Many of those who abandoned the countryside and entered the wage-dependent urban labour markets soon became desperate when they lost their jobs due to recession or ill health. Living conditions were so bad in the cities and towns, especially for the poor, that physical and mental disorders were rife. All of these factors combined to overload the workhouse system and to make a new system of separating the insane poor from the merely impoverished a priority.

2.4 THE GREAT CLIMACTERIC AND THE RISING NUMBERS OF INSANE

In 1740, the population of England was five million; by 1790 it had risen to 7.4 million, and in 1840 it was 14.8 million. Within the space of a century there were three times as many people to feed as previously. This dramatic population increase, the most notable in the history of England, is referred to as the 'great climacteric', 'climacteric' being an old medical term for a high temperature or fever. Food production and wealth generation did not keep pace with the increase in population, resulting in widespread poverty, starvation and physical and mental disease. At the beginning of the 19th century, in 1810, there were 10 701 paupers living in the city of Birmingham, the cradle of the Industrial Revolution.

The first House of Commons Select Committee to investigate the lunacy problem reported in 1807.[1] It found that there were 2248 identified insane persons in England and Wales at the beginning of that year, an incidence of 2.26 cases per 10 000 of the population. The Report considered these figures to be modest and 'scarcely a rate calculated to produce anxiety'. Their accuracy is, however, questionable. In 1805, Dr Powell had estimated the number of insane at 1 in 2000, and in 1829, Sir Andrew Halliday was to detail it as 1 in 769 or 16 000 sufferers (Jones, 1955). The Select Committee's Report led to the County Asylums Act (1808) which recommended the provision of public asylums and advised the patients in private institutions to remove to these. The Act identified four classes of patients to be provided for:

1. 'Dangerous Lunatics' detained under the Vagrancy Act (1774).
2. 'Criminal Lunatics' detained at His Majesty's pleasure under the first Criminal Lunatics Act (1800).
3. 'Pauper Lunatics' in workhouses.
4. Non-pauper or paying patients.

In its introduction, the Act stated that asylums should be built:

In an airy and healthy situation . . . but such as may afford a probability of constant medical assistance.

It suggested that asylums be located outside the towns which in the early 19th century were plagued by epidemic and endemic diseases such as typhus and cholera, but still remain accessible to visiting doctors who could not be expected to travel more than a few miles on horseback or by pony and trap. The asylums were to have separate wards for male and female patients, wards for incurables, day-rooms and airing grounds for the convalescents and 'dry and airy cells for lunatics of every description'. Treatment was to be financed by the rate system and also the full cost of maintaining the institutions, caring for and clothing the patients.

Further parliamentary proceedings followed the 1808 Act; the 1815 Parliamentary Inquiry into Madhouses was particularly critical of private madhouses which it found to be often overcrowded and brutal. Violent patients were being accommodated with non-violent to the detriment of the latter, and there were not enough attendants to care for the inmates. Inadequate

---

[1]The House of Commons Select Committee (1807) held its first meeting on 23 June 1807, under the chairmanship of C. W. W. Wynn (1775–1850), who was Under-Secretary of State at the Home Department. Wynn's Act permitted the English Counties to build hospitals for their criminal and pauper lunatics. The Act urged that the asylums be large in order to save expense, but should not exceed 300 inmates. Sites were ideally to be secured in 'airy and healthy situations, with a good supply of water and which might afford the probability of the vicinity of constant medical assistance'. Wynn's Act was of great importance in establishing the principle of hospital care through the county system, but 20 years after it was passed, only nine of the 52 English Counties had built their own asylums.

admission procedures meant that persons were being detained whose state of mind did not warrant restraint. There was generally a severe shortage of medical care and a lack of regular official visits to supervise the private madhouses' activities.

The 1844 Report of the Metropolitan Commissioners in Lunacy confirmed that a rapid rise in the total of insane persons had taken place and that the number of afflicted was almost six times that reported in 1807. In less than 30 years, insanity amongst those not able to afford a private madhouse had become a serious social problem. The Report therefore concluded that it was high time to address the problem of funding properly built asylums on a national scale.

2.5 THE 1845 LUNACY ACT AND THE ADVENT OF THE ASYLUM SYSTEM

Parliamentary and media activity repeatedly brought the problems of insanity to the fore during the 19th century. This climate of increased awareness was partly responsible for the 1845 Lunacy Act and the asylum system to which it gave birth. Digby (1985) argues that the asylum system was not simply the product of necessity borne out of overcrowding in the workhouses, but also of this heightening of public awareness. There had been a shift in public thinking about madness; by the end of the 18th century, it had come to be seen less as a spiritual disease of possession by devils, and more as a secular condition with economic repercussions. Doerner points to the significance of the work ethic:

Removing the pauper insane from the community into institutions had practical utility in freeing others in their families from caring for them and thus allowing them to work. It also underlined the values of bourgeois society where rationality came to be identified with work and irrationality with idleness and poverty. (Doerner, 1981)

Between 1844 and 1860, the population increased by just over 20% but the number of lunatics nearly doubled. By 1890, there were 86 067 officially certified cases in England and Wales, an incidence of 29.6 per 10 000 population. Even these figures were questioned by contemporary authorities. Bucknill and Tuke (1858) were sceptical of the methods used to derive them and questioned the reliability of any attempt to estimate the number of insane people. Scull (1982) considers that the amount of insanity in the country was deliberately falsified in order to allay public fear which was being fuelled by journalism of the sort found in *The Times* of 5 April 1877:

If lunacy continues to increase as at present, the insane will be in the majority and freeing themselves, will put the sane in asylums.

Concern was generated about maintaining the physical stock of the nation. If the mentally ill were allowed to breed, their children would weaken the nation's physical and mental stamina. Such an idea was in keeping with the principles of eugenics, a term coined by Francis Galton in 1883 for the attempted improvement of mankind through the adoption of genetic policies. The Eugenics Movement favoured a negative eugenics approach whereby certain categories of people, amongst them the mentally ill, would be encouraged not to have children.

The Lunacy Act, passed on 4 August 1845, heralded a new era in the care of psychiatric patients. Lord Shaftesbury, the great humanitarian reformer, was one of the architects of the Act, urging that a radical reorganization of care of the mentally ill was required. For 40 years, Shaftesbury chaired the English Lunacy Commissioners and was chief spokesperson for the Lunacy Reform Movement. He supported the idea of a comprehensive asylum system to replace the haphazard mixture of private madhouses, public workhouses, prisons and other institutions currently incarcerating mental patients. He was an admirer of what Dr Connolly had achieved at the Hanwell Asylum where mental patients were cared for without the use of chains or other means of restraint. Restraint, Shaftesbury argued, demeaned both the patient and the person who administered it. He felt that a properly administered asylum system would foster non-restraint and told his fellow parliamentarians:

> You can prevent, by the agency which you shall appoint, as you have in so many instances prevented, the recurrence of frightful cruelties: you can soothe the days of the incurable, and restore many sufferers to health and usefulness. (Hammond and Hammond, 1939)

In his speeches on the subject of new provision for the mentally ill, Shaftesbury repeatedly made reference to 'patients', 'hospitals', 'doctors' and 'nurses', apparently equating the proposed asylum system with a hospital system and implying that mental and physical illnesses were largely similar. These references to hospital personnel were at variance with Shaftesbury's proclaimed desire to provide for the mentally ill therapeutic environments based on the treatment regimens in use at the Retreat in York. The Retreat opened in 1796 and was inspired by the principles of the Quaker religion. What was on offer to patients there was not a medical approach to their mental conditions, but a philosophy of care which was quite antagonistic to medicine. The Tuke family which funded the Retreat at its inception was strongly opposed to the medical fraternity after witnessing the degrading treatment accorded to one of their own number while a patient at the York Asylum. At the Retreat, patients were treated at all times and whatever their state with respect; they were conversed with by civilized attendants and taken for long walks to expose them to the healing influences of nature. Dietary modifications were greatly favoured. Shaftesbury's thinking about new provision for the mentally ill was therefore contradictory; on the one hand, he tried to improve the status of mental patients by committing them to the care of the medical profession; on the other, as a great reformer himself, he was able to recognize and sympathize with the practices of the Retreat and wanted to see them adopted on a national scale.

Shaftesbury's vision of better care for the mentally ill had probably been modified by intensive lobbying from senior members of the medical profession who had certainly not been slow to see the possibilities of turning an asylum system into a means of increasing the power of doctors. Psychiatry would have an institutional base in which to consolidate and then expand its activities. Utilizing public paranoia to its own advantage, the medical profession began claiming to be able to identify people who might become insane, to treat them when they did become mad and finally to return them to society fit for work. Where workhouses had been a totally inappropriate environment for medical aspirations to scientific respectability, doctors saw that asylums could be places not only of reform but also of treatment, in all ways resembling the general hospitals in which they, as doctors, were already entrenched.

The interest and concern of a few humanitarians and politicians brought the mentally ill onto the political agenda at the beginning of the 19th century. Their enthusiasm resulted in the creation of a revolutionary new system of care based in asylums. However, the political pioneers paid little attention to practical matters surrounding the costs of such a system, or the numbers and kind of personnel who would be required to staff it. The medical profession therefore found itself with a *carte blanche* to implement its supposedly scientific treatments when it moved into the asylums. Connolly (1830) foresaw immense difficulties arising from the strategy of dealing with the insane by removing them from their everyday environments and incarcerating them with large numbers of other insane people, to the exacerbation of everyone's madness. Nor had any thought been given to the role of the attendants who were going to deliver medically ordained care to the patients and the attendants therefore found themselves moving into uncharted territory when they started to offer mass care to institutionalized patients under the authority of medical superintendents. In the next chapters, an account will be offered of how psychiatric nursing developed from the early years of the asylum system, when a basis for and philosophy of care were being created, to the present day. Nurses are to be viewed not from the standpoint of their political or medical masters, but, as far as historical resources will allow, are to be heard speaking for themselves.

REFERENCES

Bucknill, J. C. and Tuke, D. H. (1858) *A Manual of Psychological Medicine*, Blanchard and Lee, Philadelphia.

Clarke, B. (1975) *Mental Disorder in Early Britain*, University of Wales Press, Cardiff.

Connolly, J. (1830) *An Inquiry Concerning the Indications of Insanity with Suggestions for the Better Protection and Care of the Insane*, Taylor, London.

Cowper, W. (1816) *Memoirs of the Early Life of William Cowper Esq.*, R. Edwards, London, p. 27.

Digby, A. (1985) *Madness, Morality and Medicine: a study of the York Retreat*, Cambridge University Press, Cambridge.

Doerner, K. (1981) Introduction, in *Madmen and the Bourgeoisie*, Basil Blackwell, Oxford.

Foucault, M. (1965) *Madness and Civilisation*, Tavistock, London.

Hammond, J. L. and Hammond, B. (1939) *Lord Shaftesbury*, Penguin Books, London, p. 195.

Haslam, J. (1809) *Observations on Madness and Melancholy*, 2nd edn, J. Callow, London, p. 26.

Henriques, U. (1979) *Before the Welfare State*, Longman, London, p. 14.

Hunter, R. and Macalpine, I. (1970) *Three Hundred Years of Psychiatry*, Oxford University Press, London.

Hunter, R. and Macalpine, I. (1974) *Psychiatry for the Poor*, Dawsons of Pall Mall.

Jones, K. (1955) *Lunacy, Law and Conscience 1744–1845*, Routledge & Kegan Paul, London.

Jones, W. L. (1983) *Ministering to Minds Diseased – A History of Psychiatric Treatment*, William Heinemann Medical Books Ltd., London.

Purcell, M. (1982) *A Time for Sowing – The History of St. John of God Brothers in Ireland 1879–1979*, Hospitaller Brothers of St. John of God, Dublin.

Scull, A. (1982) *Museums of Madness*, Penguin Books, London, p. 18.

Tate, W. E. (1969) *The Parish Chest*, Cambridge University Press, Cambridge, p. 72.

Walk, A. (1961) The history of mental nursing. *Journal of Mental Science*, **107**, 1–17.

3

Asylum care and culture

3.1 INTRODUCTION

Before examining who the 19th century attendants were and what they did, it is important to have an appreciation of the context in which they worked. This context includes contemporary classifications of mental disorder and ideas about its treatment and medical and social expectations of what attendant care should be.

3.2 DEFINITIONS OF INSANITY IN THE MID–19TH CENTURY

Social attitudes towards people with mental disorders have always influenced the quality of care which they have received. When looking at psychiatry in the 19th century, and at the state of the art of mental nursing, it is important to understand what theories about mental illness and what prejudices those caring for the mentally sick brought with them to their work. Poverty was just beginning to be understood in England as a cause of mental disease. During the great climacteric, there had been a rapid increase in population and a parallel increase in poverty. The significance of poverty in the epidemiology of disease, the connection between bad living conditions, ill health and unhappiness had been forcibly expressed most notably by Friederich Engels (1969). He wrote of the destitution caused by urbanization and of the sufferings of the poor who breathed polluted air, lived in overcrowded tenements with little sanitation, and had no access to clean water. They were the almost inevitable victims of mental disturbance:

They are exposed to the most exciting changes in mental condition, the most violent vibrations between hope and fear: they are hunted like game, and not permitted to attain peace of mind and quiet enjoyment of life. They are deprived of all enjoyments except that of sexual indulgence and drunkenness, are worked every day to the point of complete exhaustion of their mental and physical energies, and are thus constantly spurred on to the maddest excess in the only two enjoyments at their disposal. (Engels, 1969)

Alongside the social theories of madness existed ideas centring on the new discoveries about genetics. *Inheritance theory* held that insanity, like other ailments, could be transmitted from one generation to the next. Other authorities espoused the theory of *moral degeneracy* and considered that the sufferings of a certain percentage of those who were poor and ill were due simply to badness of character. These 'criminal lunatics' were considered unreformable. On the whole, poverty was not to be seen as an excuse for crime. White (1885), writing in the 1880s, divided the poor into three categories: 20% genuinely unemployed; 40% feckless and incapable; 40% wholly degenerate. As far as the 80% 'physically, mentally and morally unfit' were concerned:

There is nothing that the nation can do for them except to let them die out by leaving them alone. (White, 1885).

From the inheritance and moral degeneracy theories sprang the Eugenics Movement which was strongly influenced by Darwin, Spencer and Francis Galton, and which held that if a genetically and morally inferior section of society was allowed to propagate freely, it would within a short space of time outnumber the rest of society. Allowing such poor quality individuals to reproduce would reverse the course of evolution, returning human civilization to an animal state. Eugenicists recommended that measures should be taken to detect and isolate people likely to become insane, and to segregate them so as to prevent their breeding. Society must be made 'secure from their degradation and danger of their propagation' (Tredgold, 1909). Adherents of the Eugenics Movement frequently referred their British audiences to the position in Ireland, where, they claimed, hundreds of defectives were being allowed freely to reproduce, leading to degeneracy on a massive scale! Connolly Norman, a leading Irish psychiatrist of the early 1900s, presented what he considered 'proof' that 'feeble-minded people produced rather larger numbers of children than did the sound-minded' (Finnane, 1991). His conclusion, therefore, was that to enforce birth control on the feeble-minded would act to reduce insanity if not eradicate it completely.

In asylums where such ideas prevailed, patients were seen as degenerates and staff had instructions to guard against associations between male and female patients. Nor were the staff themselves considered trustworthy as male and female attendants were also kept apart! The superintendent assumed responsibility for the morals of his attendants who, if they went outside of the institution on their day off, had to inform him of what they intended to do and who they were going to see. Staff had to seek permission to marry, and in the case of females, were obliged to resign on marrying. Married men still had to live in on the wards and went home only on their days off. Such measures suggest that some superintendents viewed their employees as no 'better' than the patients.

Miasmic theory was based on the assumption that dirt and putrefaction were the principal causes of bad health in mind and body. Putrefaction gave rise to smells which carried disease-causing organisms. Diseased people themselves gave off smells which could then contaminate others (Goldstein, 1984). Miasmic theory allowed the middle and upper classes to believe that it must be the poor who were most at risk of illness and most dangerous to the health to the rest of society. In asylums where superintendents subscribed to this theory, there was a preoccupation with hygiene. Walls were white-washed and floors were scrubbed several times a day. Staff not only super-vised the bathing of individuals, but diligently recorded their weight, general health, the state of their toe nails and finger nails, any marks or scars on their body and whether they had lice.

Those who favoured the **contagion theory** of illness, also referred to as the **germ theory**, believed that the vectors for disease were not smells but individuals. Patients were therefore managed on the principle which Arm-strong (1983) has referred to as 'sanitizing social space'. They were categorized and segregated according to their conditions on the supposition that segre-gation would prevent others from becoming infected. It was also believed that bringing patients into the open air could prevent the spread of illness. Therefore, those patients who were too frail to work would spend long periods walking each day in the airing courts or be brought outside on their beds. Each ward had its own airing court separated from others by a high wall.

Other theories of mental illness also found favour during the 19th century. Vitamin C deficiency was thought to be the cause of a condition known as 'haematoma auris', a blood clot in the middle ear and regarded as a sign of degeneration. Some doctors favoured the **septic foci theory** of insanity and would operate on patients to remove what they thought was the source of their infection and hence their insanity, e.g. their teeth, tonsils or parts of the gastric tract. The 'Simian Hand' was described in the literature until well into the 20th century, the hands of some patients being thought to resemble an ape's, indicative of dementia praecox (Hunter and Macalpine, 1974).

It does not appear that the attendants as a group espoused any one of these theories in preference to the others. The views of their particular superintendent and of the doctors who worked at their asylum were the most important in influencing their thinking. Some who read the *Journal of Mental Science* would have been aware of wider ideas about the causation of mental illness, and would perhaps have passed on their knowledge to colleagues.

3.3 CLASSIFICATION OF MENTAL DISORDERS

One of the earliest attempts to classify patients according to their conditions was undertaken at the Lancashire Asylum during the 1850s. Ten wards

Table 3.1 Conditions suffered by patients admitted to Rainhill during 1860

Moral cause	Males	Females
Disappointment	2	0
Grief	9	7
Religious excitement	8	6
Fright	1	2
Unfounded charges against character	0	1
Jealousy	0	1
Excitement	1	0
Embarrassment	3	0
Poverty	2	6
Disappointment in love	0	1
Anxiety	0	1

Source: Rainhill Admission Register (1860).

were designated for different generic categories of patient. By 1860, these categories had become so well established that they appeared in the asylum's Annual Report. The various categories show the types of patients that attendants were caring for (source: The Rainhill Asylum Admission Register, 1860).

1. Dementia cases: described as active, orderly and quiet patients who had been some time in the institution and were capable of rendering assistance in other cases of dementia.
2. Recent cases: described as active, orderly and quiet patients who had been some time in the institution and who could assist with other cases recently admitted.
3. Non-violent, non-suicidal and non-escapees.
4. Convalescents.
5. Refractory and excited cases.
6. Suicidal, associated with cheerful and watchful cases.
7. Refractory and violent epileptics.
8. Non-violent epileptics.
9. Aged quiet cases.
10. Infirmary.

Rainhill Asylum further divided its patients into 'moral' and 'physical' categories depending on where the origin of their condition was thought to lie. The type of categorization employed at Rainhill was frequently referred to and discussed in the *Journal of Mental Science* and it must therefore be assumed that its use was widespread.

Patients with the conditions shown in Table 3.1 were admitted to Rainhill during 1860.

'Grief' and 'religious excitement' account for the largest number of patients admitted and yet the history of psychiatric care has little to say about the

Table 3.2 Physical causes for insanity

Physical cause	Males	Females
Epilepsy	10	11
Injury to the head	6	0
Intemperance	6	5
Scrofula	1	0
Working with paint	1	0
Vicious practices	1	0
Hard study	1	0
Imprisonment	1	0
Rheumatic fever	1	0
Brain disease	1	0
Disability after parturition	0	3
Pregnancy	0	1
Overwork	0	1
Climactic change	0	1
Affection of uterus	0	1
Paralysis	0	1
Disability after illness	0	1
Exposure to vicissitudes of climate	0	1
Congenital	5	6
Hereditary	3	3
Unknown	51	111

Source: Rainhill Admission Register (1860).

treatments that these patients were supposed to receive. In practice, in the absence of established treatment regimes, it was left to the discretion of the attendants as to how the patients were managed. It appears that what treatments there were were administered *en masse* with little variation according to individual cases.

Physical causes for insanity were described at Rainhill as shown in Table 3.2.

The fact that most patients admitted were categorized as being ill due to 'unknown causes' reflects the contemporary state of the diagnostic art in psychiatry. It may also reflect the honesty of asylum doctors who, unlike their descendants of the late 20th century, did not feel under pressure to give scientific names to conditions of which they had little understanding. Despite, or perhaps because of the large numbers classified as suffering from 'unknown causes', there was a high discharge rate. Much has been written about the harshness of the conditions in the asylums, yet many patients apparently improved sufficiently to be discharged home 'cured'. In 1860, the Prestwich Asylum recorded the figures shown in Table 3.3 for length of stay.

The longer the patients remained in hospital, the less likely they were to be discharged. In 1860, 64 patients at Prestwich were discharged within one year of their admission and, of these, 29 had stayed for less than 3 months. The total number of patients in the asylum in 1860 was 502, giving a discharge

Table 3.3 Duration of stay of patients discharged cured

Duration	Males	Females	Total
Under 3 months	13	16	29
Under 6 months	5	10	15
Under 9 months	8	6	14
Under 12 months	2	4	6
Under 18 months	2	3	5
Under 2 years	1	2	3
Under 3 years	2	3	5
Under 4 years	0	1	1
Under 5 years	0	0	0
Under 6 years	0	1	1
Under 9 years	0	1	1
Total	33	47	80

Source: Prestwich Asylum Annual Report (1860).

rate of 13% for that year, a rate which remained constant throughout the decade. The diagnoses of those discharged were as shown in Table 3.4.

3.4 MORAL MANAGEMENT

The new keenness manifest in the first half of the 19th century to survey the practices of caring for the insane was partly due to an awakening of public consciousness and partly to a new spirit of management. Walk (1961) explains that 'moral management', as it was known, attempted to replace the traditional reliance on mechanical restraints for controlling patients with non-physical methods. It was not a philosophy which was embraced nationally. Parry-Jones (1972) claims that only those superintendents who ran private high-class madhouses supported it. In these institutions, money could buy civility; those who opposed moral management were superintendents of poorly resourced asylums for pauper lunatics. These men saw moral management as a soft option, believing it would encourage patients to remain idle and insane. Their spokesperson was William Cullen (1710–1790), a distinguished Edinburgh medical teacher:

Table 3.4 Cures with respect to the form of insanity in 1860

Diagnosis	Cures		
	Males	Females	Total
Mania	23	27	50
Mania puerperal	–	2	2
Melancholia	5	12	17
Dementia	5	6	11
Total	33	47	80

Source: Prestwich Asylum Annual Report (1860).

Restraining the anger and violence of madmen is always necessary for preventing their hurting themselves or others; but this restraint is also to be considered as a remedy. Angry passions are always rendered more violent by the indulgence of the impetuous motions they produce; and even in madmen, the feeling of restraint will sometimes prevent the efforts which their passions would otherwise occasion. Restraint therefore is useful and ought to be complete. (Cullen, 1780)

Cullen considered the insane as akin to wild animals whose spirit had to be broken in order to uphold the supremacy of reason. When he and men like him appointed attendants, they favoured tall, strong and disciplined individuals, well able to impose restraint. Dr Samuel Hadwin of the Lincoln Asylum saw restraint as a means of therapy:

Restraint forms the very basis and principle on which the sound treatment of lunatics is founded. The judicious and appropriate adaptation of the various modifications of this powerful means to the peculiarities of each case of insanity comprises a large portion of the curative regimen of the scientific and rational practitioner; in his hands, it is a remedial agent of the finest importance. (Hadwin, 1985)

Some superintendents resisted moral management on financial grounds, claiming that to employ enough servants for the care of inmates who 'were not ironed' would entail a larger expenditure than they could afford. In their turn, many attendants were nervous of abandoning the use of physical restraint because they felt it would lead to more patients escaping for which the staff would be penalized. At Duddeston Hall, one of the rules read as follows:

Any nurse or servant from whose custody a patient escapes through negligence, shall pay the expense of retaking the patient. (Rule Book, Duddeston Hall, Warwickshire)

Restraint was also enlisted on the side of moral reform, being generally seen as an acceptable form of treatment for those considered to have let their passions have free reign.

There were practical problems facing those who wanted to abolish physical means of restraint. Severe overcrowding in the asylums meant that even where restraint was not used, seclusion and solitary confinement had often to replace it as a necessary form of controlling refractory patients. Many superintendents of public asylums and proprietors of private madhouses brought into use padded cells for violent patients.

There was a danger also that the public's conscience concerning the welfare of mental patients would be lulled by the adoption of non-restraint when, in essence, attitudes towards the mentally ill had not changed at all. John Connolly wrote on this point to *The Times* on 10 December 1840:

> More actual cruelty [is] hidden under the show of humanity in the system of non-coercion than is openly displayed in muffs, strait-waistcoats, leg-locks and coercion chairs.

Dr Mundy, who travelled extensively, visiting asylums in Britain and Europe, noted the gap between what Lunacy Reform had promised and what was being delivered:

> I must with pain confess that a model asylum does not exist . . . and that the lunatic asylums of Europe are still in a very unsatisfactory condition, whilst the number of those suited to their purpose form only a small exception. (Mundy, 1861)

The great disparity between how the wealthy insane and the poor were treated frequently spurred Mundy to fury. He contrasted the comfortable surroundings of some asylums which were tastefully furnished and well provided with books and journals and where patients were cared for by polite and cultured servants, with the miserable conditions too often endured by poor patients. In the worst asylums, the atmosphere was prison-like. There was a total absence of stimulation; indeed, some patients spent their days in airless cells without light. Bedding was primitive and no heating provided even in the severest winters, resulting in a high rate of deaths from hypothermia.

The majority of institutions, according to Mundy, fell between these two extremes. For the most part, asylums were akin to small manufacturing towns where self-sufficiency was a guiding principle, and to keep the patients usefully occupied was the foremost duty of the staff:

> They had there special shops for smiths, locksmiths, turners, house-painters, upholsterers, cabinet makers, book-binders, etc. and not infrequently printers are found who execute all the printing for the establishment; whilst brewers, bakers, butchers, and millers carry on their several occupations in the particular departments allotted to them and supply the wants of the asylum . . . the other sex are engaged in the delicate work of ladies, such as embroidery, whilst others are occupied with the hard work of the washhouse, ironing, cleaning and with the business of the kitchen or with housekeeping; whilst others again are industriously engaged in needle-work and knitting. (Mundy, 1861)

Mundy concluded that the needs of the individual patients were subordinate to the superintendents' desire to keep the asylum self-sufficient and preferably, profitable. Yet they were, Mundy reminded the Medico-Psychological

Association, supposed to be doctors running hospitals, and not managers running businesses.

Mundy found the status of 'psychological physicians' to be generally low and was interested to find out why this was so. There was on average only one doctor to every 300 lunatics and his salary was meagre in comparison to that received by doctors working in other branches of medicine. Mundy noted that doctors, and especially the proprietors of private asylums, cloaked their establishments in secrecy, giving the impression to the public at large that shameful and frightening doings were afoot behind the closed doors.

3.5 THE ASYLUM SYSTEM, SOCIETY AND THE MEDICAL PROFESSION

The emergence of the asylum system reflected the increasing power of the State over the lives of individuals in the mid–19th century. Although the asylums wrapped their aims in medical rhetoric, as state-funded institutions their purpose was essentially social and lay in welfare administration. Baldwin (1971) sees powerful political and economic forces behind the growth of the asylum system. Its justification on moral grounds – bringing medical aid to deranged and powerless people – was always weak because the total disrespect for the freedom of the individual which the system embodied tended to contradict its appeal to humanitarianism. Those idealists who had hoped that the newly built institutions would be **hospitals** where mentally ill patients could be protected from the hostility of society, were rapidly disillusioned:

> Those worthy aims were thwarted by the very size of the problem they sought to master, leading to the self-strangulation of the mental institution as a hospital and its replacement by the crowded, stagnant, medically important asylum. (Baldwin, 1971)

Scull (1982) finds his explanation for the birth of the asylum system in the attitude of 19th century humanitarians whom he considers were principally upper class Evangelicals and Benthamites. Scull is suspicious of their motives, regarding their attitudes as self-righteous and their outlook as that of a dominant class towards those lower down the social structure. Evangelical rhetoric, he finds, may have concealed class interests. It was a:

> conservative movement, concerned to shore up a disintegrating social structure and paternalistic morality against the threats posed by an undisciplined lower class rabble and by a purely maternalistic entrepreneurial class. (Scull, 1982)

It was satisfactory to the influential part of Victorian society to see destitution controlled by the removal of pauper lunatics into asylums. There the indigent became a witness to the State's humanity; they were provided with food, medicines, recreation and even free burials should they die. (It should be observed, however, that the provision of food failed to prevent patients from starving as humanitarianism did not entirely override the long-held belief that the poor should not be overfed for fear of their becoming soft and indolent.) In return for their keep, the recipients of welfare were expected to be grateful and subservient. They were to be taught the necessity of leading an ordered existence and their spiritual needs, which it was presumed they must have neglected, were to be catered for by daily services and preaching.

Working hand in glove with the State in the establishment of the asylums was the medical profession, keen to carve out a prime place for itself within the newly emerging branch of medicine which was to become known as psychiatry. Doctors presented the asylum system in a package attractive to the Victorian mind, suggesting that psychiatry had a major contribution to make to the national industrial advance by getting sick people back to work. Therapy was available, it was claimed, which would speed up the discharge rate, thus enabling patients to re-enter the labour market quickly. Much later, when such a claim proved difficult to meet, merely removing people from society was marketed as a medical contribution to the health of society. Those who criticized the institutions on financial grounds were reassured that within a short space of time, they would become self-financing as, in accordance with the prevalent spirit of self-help, those in receipt of treatment and care would contribute to the asylums' maintenance. By setting the institutions in extensive farm land and using patients as the labour force, they would have the means of becoming not only self-sufficient but profitable.

Doctors were largely successful in introducing a medical perspective on mental illness and its treatment, and on the care of those suffering from it. The disease model, with its claim to scientific respectability, was the approach then uniting all branches of medicine and became fundamental to thinking about mental illness (Mitchell, 1984). Such a perspective, still very much to the fore 150 years later, is directly descended from Newton's view of the body as a mechanism. All ill health is seen as a malfunction of a particular organ or part of the body. The task of the health profession is to diagnose the problem and repair the malfunctioning part. Doctors saw cure as their objective, not prevention of illness, health education or the understanding of the complex interaction of relationships affecting any individual in society. The perceived power to cure placed the medical profession firmly in the centre of the mental illness stage; doctors had created a legitimizing ideology which strongly underpinned their power and prestige.

Mitchell (1984) argues that there is a connection between the supremacy of the medical model and the relegation of nursing to a low status occupation. Because to 'cure' was the all important goal in psychiatry, 'caring' became a mere adjunct to this activity. Caring could be carried out by friends and relatives; it did not require professional expertise. It was about looking after people on the way to being 'cured' or who were unfortunately incurable.

3.6 THE ATTENDANTS

The new asylums were almost immediately overwhelmed by large numbers of ex-workhouse inmates with chronic illnesses: within a short period, over 90% of the asylum population were classified as paupers (Korman and Glennerster, 1990). The asylums were expected to be self-financing and this meant that labour costs had to be kept to a minimum. The priority for superintendents was to generate income. This was achieved in most instances by admitting as many patients as possible, particularly those from outside the asylum's catchment area, the rationale being that a standard rate was paid to the asylum for patients from within the locality, but considerably more could be negotiated for those from outside the area. The financial pressure placed on the superintendents and Boards of Governors of the asylums meant that staff were expected to undertake a wide variety of duties.

From whatever roots the asylum system sprang, it is doubtlessly true that the preoccupations of politicians and members of Boards of Asylum Governors did not centre on the attendants who were probably only marginally less considered than the patients themselves. Nonetheless, it was through the work of the attendants that psychiatry was being delivered and some interested parties were moved to look more closely at the kind of persons employed to care for and supervise patients. There were no generally agreed criteria as to what constituted a good attendant; very different types of people were selected from institution to institution, a situation which persisted until recent times. What is found in the literature, therefore, are many images of many attendants, but these attendants were all pioneers and laying down the foundations of modern psychiatric nursing.

The attendants occupied the middle ground between the doctors and the patients. Socially and intellectually, their status was considered far inferior to that of the medical staff, but their closeness to the patients made them highly influential in the patients' lives. For the most part, more was expected of the attendants than their background and lack of training made it possible for them to deliver. They represented cheap labour, and it was quite unreasonable to expect that once in contact with patients they should behave as if they were experts in looking after mentally ill people. In the majority of asylums during the 1850s and 1860s, attendants were given no training, nor was there any career structure for them. The quality of training in the few asylums which offered it varied depending on the knowledge and enthusiasm of the superintendents.

Abel-Smith (1977) considered that the attendants and nurses of the mid–19th century were generally not capable of doing the work entrusted to them. He concurred with Florence Nightingale's observations that many of those who were employed to care for the sick would not have found work elsewhere because they were too old, alcoholic or too lazy. Male attendants were commonly regarded as the 'unemployed of other professions'. Asylum work was of low status and not popular, and the stigma of the insane rubbed off on those who worked with them (Carpenter, 1980).

In the private asylum at Worcester in the early 1800s, keepers were generally recruited from the lowest social groups, although a few came from the ranks of the skilled working class. The majority were unskilled agricultural workers, whose care had hitherto been devoted to cows and pigs. By contrast, keepers at the Stafford Asylum were drawn from an urban working class with experience in shoe-making, building, gardening and glazing. Most female staff employed in asylum work had previously been in domestic service and many of the men had been in the army. Superintendents tended to look for attributes such as size and strength in potential attendants rather than for any signs of ability to relate to patients. Records suggest that in a number of asylums, staff were recruited from the ranks of ex-patients, although this was risky because such keepers tended to relapse and need readmission as patients themselves. Superintendents were probably driven to taking on ex-patients as attendants because of the problems involved in securing staff from the local labour force, and because of pressure to keep their asylums' running costs down. Some asylums devised a promotion scheme in order to incline staff to stay, such as at the Stafford Asylum where all female staff started as laundry girls, progressed to becoming housemaids, then upper housemaids and eventually, keepers! (Smith, 1988).

According to one attendant who entered the asylum service in 1852, the male attendants tended to fall into four categories (Newman, 1986). Firstly, there were those who were referred to as 'solid men' or 'stout men'. Their background was in farm labour; they were physically strong and used to hard manual work. These men were cherished by superintendents because they could contribute to the running of the asylum farms, and therefore to the income of the institution. They could also help to administer unpleasant treatments generally regarded by patients as punishments. To subject patients to the 'bath of surprise', cold showers, or the swivel chair took a considerable amount of strength which the farm-labourer attendants could provide. However, keeping these workers proved difficult because they were easily tempted away to more lucrative agricultural work. Farm attendants at the Lancaster Asylum stayed for an average of only 15 months.

Secondly, there were those workers whose families had been connected with the workhouse system for many years, institutional work being carried on from one generation to the next. Superintendents often asked those whom they considered good employees if they had any children or relatives who might be interested in working at the asylum. They knew that staff children brought up close to the asylum would have realistic expectations of the work and would be supervised and advised by their parents.

Next, those who had been in service to the gentry as butlers, footmen, gardeners or labourers frequently took work in asylums. They were used to taking orders and to working long hours for little pay. The last and smallest category of male attendants comprised ex-servicemen from the army and navy. These men were much liked by superintendents because of their disciplined background and their ability both to lead and be led.

Attendants' pay was very low: in the early days of the asylum system, between 3 and 4 shillings a week, depending on the price of the local labour market. The average weekly wage for a farm labourer at this time was about 15 shillings a week. The comparison is not strictly accurate, however, because asylum staff also received full board, a uniform and periodic entertainment. Their official hours of duty were from 6.00 a.m to 10.00 p.m., but in reality they could be called on 24 hours a day.

The records of Littlemore Asylum show the rates of pay (per annum) for different grades of staff in 1863 (source: Annual Report for Littlemore Asylum, 1863).

Superintendent	£450
Medical assistant	£100
Chaplain	£180
Clerk of visitors	£126
Treasurer	£30
Auditor	£37/10
Clerk of asylum	£120
Housekeeper	£40
Head male attendant	£40
Head female attendant	£25
Head female laundry attendant	£25
Male attendant	£20–£25
Female attendant	£14–£18

Superintendents' desire to maximize on the skills of their attendants in order to increase the viability of their asylum is demonstrated in the arrangements at the Worcester County Asylum:

Most of the attendants are artisans who work with the patients, do all the repairs and anything requiring attention. The shoemaker takes chief charge of the 1st Male Convalescent Ward as well as overseeing the shoe-repair shop. The mason takes charge of the 2nd Convalescent Ward: he is glazier, painter and decorator. The tailor assists in the 4th or Epileptic Ward at meal-times and in the evenings. The 5th Ward has two attendants: the junior takes charge of the barrow men and assists in all excavations and wheeling of earth. It is only by such arrangements that any asylum can be conducted efficiently. (Medical Report of the Worcester County Asylum, 1851)

The diary of an attendant first employed at the Wiltshire Asylum in 1852 details how he came to work there and the problems he encountered when he wanted to get married (Newman, 1986, personal communication). He was interviewed by the superintendent, Dr Thurnam, and selected because he was a skilled man, by trade a master-tailor, and a Christian. He was 26 years old when he started at the asylum and his work consisted of making clothes for patients and staff and teaching some patients the art of tailoring. His official title was attendant-tailor.

The woman he married was employed as a domestic servant to Dr Thurnam and his wife and her status was in fact superior to his although she earned less than he did. The attendant asked permission of his superintendent to marry as was the practice, but when Dr Thurnam discovered that the bride to be was his own servant, 'he was not at all pleased'! Eventually he agreed, but banned the wedding until he had found a suitable replacement for his lost maid. This girl was never in paid employment again, and her husband was required to live in on the wards for 10 years after their marriage, visiting her only on his days off. After this period, he was allowed to live out!

The majority of asylums, like the general hospitals, referred to female attendants as 'nurses'. Nurses were drawn mainly from those who would otherwise have gone into domestic service (Newman, 1986, personal communication). For young women, the attraction of the job lay in its providing full board and lodging, but the work was harder than service to the gentry and the only social life they could look forward to was going home on their days off, or meeting, at infrequent intervals, some of the male attendants. In the event of their marrying, they lost their posts. Male and female attendants were required to remain in their own areas of the asylum and mixed only on rare sporting and social occasions when their interaction was strictly supervised.

Older women who went into asylum nursing were either widows or married women who had brought up their families and now wished for some independence. This older group made up the majority of the nurses. No particular skills were required of them other than being able to cope with long hours and hard work. Older women were preferred by superintendents because they were already accustomed to hard work and did not complain about their conditions of service. They were also unlikely to leave to have babies or get married.

3.7 ATTENDANTS IN THE MEDICAL LITERATURE

The term 'psychiatry' was first used in England in 1846 by asylum doctors keen to christen and so have acknowledged this newly emerging branch of medicine. The Medico-Psychological Association (MPA) was founded at the instigation of Dr Samuel Hitch in 1841. Dr Hitch was the resident superintendent at the Gloucester Lunatic Asylum and the first meeting of the Association was held there. In attendance were Dr Gaskell (Lancaster Asylum), Dr Shute (Gloucester Asylum), Dr Powell (Nottingham Asylum), Dr Thurnam (the Retreat, York) and Mr Wintle (Oxford Asylum). The Association began to publish its own journal in 1853 which was initially entitled *The Asylum Journal*, but soon became known as the *Journal of Mental Science*. Its circulation was confined to the new county asylums built as a result of the 1845 Act, but it helped to establish the credibility of psychiatry as a branch of medical science. Through the Journal, young aspiring doctors acquired ideas and disseminated their own.

Although the content of the earlier issues was aimed mostly at doctors, there was also subject matter of interest to other asylum workers. The Journal attempted to be truly multidisciplinary. Jobs of all grades were advertised. For example, an 'experienced cook' was wanted in Devon at the rate of £20 per annum. A 'clinical assistant' was needed in Oxfordshire at a rate of £70 per annum plus board. A Medical Superintendent was sought for the Worcester Asylum after the suicide of Dr Grahamsley; this post offered £350 per annum, furnished accommodation, coals, candles and vegetables from the garden. There was also information in the Journal about various aspects of the work of the attendant. Certain doctors were to be found advocating better conditions for attendants and nurses. From the start of the asylum system, doctors had assumed responsibility for the selection, supervision and termination of employment of attendants, realizing that the success of the system was heavily dependent on them.

Dr Kirkbride, an honorary member of the MPA in its early years, and Physician-in-Chief at the Pennsylvania Hospital for the Insane in Philadelphia, was a prodigious writer for the Journal. He travelled regularly to England where he had many friends who were superintendents. Dr Kirkbride set great store by the asylum attendants and his views were esteemed by his colleagues. Because of his considerable reputation on both sides of the Atlantic, his writings on and for the attendants are of special interest. As early as 1841, he prepared a *Manual for Attendants* in which he spelt out the requirements of a 'good attendant':

> A high moral character, a good education, strict temperance, kind and respectful manners, a cheerful and forbearing temper, with calmness under irritation, industry, zeal and watchfulness in the discharge of duty, and above all that sympathy which springs from the heart, are among the qualities which are desirable. (Tuke, 1884)

He was forced to acknowledge that finding such upright individuals to work in the asylums was not easy. In addition to selecting attendants who could carry out the everyday duties involved in running the institution, Kirkbride felt that there was also a need for a limited number of attendants of a 'high order' who could be released from the ordinary ward tasks in order to devote their full attention to patients:

> If properly qualified, no persons can add more essentially to the comfort and happiness of the insane than the attendants. (Tuke, 1884)

In 1861, Kirkbride was urging the MPA to give serious consideration to the training of attendants. He argued that patients would so benefit from being cared for by a trained attendant that their stay in hospital would be considerably reduced.

When considering nursing for the insane, Dr Mundy insisted that psychiatry could not become established and respected unless the people chosen to care for the insane were men and women of ability and compassion. Like Kirkbride, he felt that the standards expected of attendants must be the same as those expected of nurses in general hospitals. It was of concern to him that the status of psychiatry and of mental nursing was being dragged down by carers of the worst sort and he singled out for special condemnation the religious fraternities who looked after mental patients. In their institutions, Mundy found that perverted and impractical ideas were rife; restraint flourished and barbarities were conducted that would have been considered out of place in bygone ages. In general, Mundy felt that the numbers of attendants were much too small and considered:

> Their character and qualifications leave very much to be desired. Their salaries and future provision are lamentably insufficient, and we have not yet arrived at the recognition of the necessity of schools for the education of attendants. (Mundy, 1861)

Maudsley also felt that attendants and particularly women attendants should be more highly valued:

> An elderly female nurse of a kind and sensible disposition, could not fail to be a great comfort to those patients who require gentle and sympathetic attention, and might be expected often to exert a very beneficial influence over them. Assuredly some would yield to women's persuasion more readily and with less feeling of humiliation then to the dictates of an attendant of their own sex. (Maudsley, 1879)

Dr Crichton Browne of the West Riding Asylum implemented Maudsley's idea. He selected a nurse, the wife of one of his attendants, and placed her on a 70-bed ward for epileptic and suicidal patients. She apparently transformed the ward so that it became quieter and more orderly. To Browne's mind, a mixture of male and female staff could make unruly male wards as calm as the female wards. His own experiment was, however, confined to one ward, and was very much the exception rather than the rule in asylums generally.

3.8 INTERPRETATIONS OF THE WORK OF THE ATTENDANT

In the early days of the asylums, the attendants' role was not clearly defined. Every superintendent stamped his own personality on the institution he ran, and laid down what he wanted his attendants to do. There was no body of knowledge on which to base a coherent system of care and treatment. Some superintendents saw the attendants as obedient servants of the institution; others saw them primarily as servants to the patients; others again saw the role of the attendant as that of a spiritual guide. There was also the view that the attendants were simply intermediaries between doctors and patients.

3.8.1 The Attendant as Rule-Keeper and Enforcer

A *Rule Book* was issued to each attendant when he took up his asylum duties and rule-keeping was considered of primary importance. If he transgressed, he might be dismissed; equally it was his duty to enforce the rules appertaining to the patients. It would appear that even though the superintendants claimed to want 'higher class persons' to come forward as attendants, they did little to recruit such people, preferring, in fact, those with less initiative and independence of spirit who would readily conform to the asylums' regimes.

3.8.2 The Attendant as Servant to the Patients

There had been attendants waiting on patients since the beginning of the 18th century. At that time, in the well-managed, private madhouses owned by clergymen or doctors which targeted their services at the wealthy, the patients were cared for in comfortable surroundings and by servants whose job it was to minister to their every need. Treatment consisted mainly in exposing the patients to civilized company and behaviour. Some 19th century superintendents subscribed, at least in principle, to this role for their attendants, although there is no confirmation in the literature that any of them ever realized it in practice. Dr John Connolly believed that the influence of the attendant over the patient was considerable and suggested that such highly skilled individuals undermined their own position by failing to demand better working conditions than those they commonly endured (Connolly, 1847).

3.8.3 The Attendant as Spiritual Guide

Some superintendents who had been influenced by the Quaker-inspired Moral Management Movement saw the attendant as a spiritual guide, demonstrating in his work the practical application of Christian principles. Men such as Jepson believed in and practised spiritual healing and considered attendants and doctors as mere instruments in a healing process brought about by God. One of the early Quaker superintendents, John Thurnam, who took from the Retreat at York its Quaker ideology and replanted it at his Wiltshire Asylum, believed in exposing his patients to nature through walks and sport and through the cultivation of the institution's beautiful grounds. He felt that men and women encountered God in the natural world where He manifested Himself. Thurnam's attendants were led to believe that they were channels for God's divine powers of curing the sick. This attitude was echoed in Florence Nightingale's words:

> What nursing has to do . . . is put the patient in the best condition for nature to act upon him. (Nightingale, 1863)

Once at peace with his God, the mentally ill patient was then ready to be healed. The attendant's duty was to bring about and then sustain that inward peace.

3.8.4 The Attendant as Intermediary between Doctor and Patient

In some asylums, the hidden curriculum appeared to be that attendants should stand guard at the boundaries between rational society and the chaotic world of the mentally ill, between high status doctors and uncivilized patients. The attendants protected the medical authorities from the contamination of patients:

> Thus insulated from the reality of asylum existence, the superintendent was able to remain a remote, if benevolent despot, his position above the crowd and freedom from too close and frequent contact with the patients protecting him from contamination not just of his social position, but, indirectly, of his authority as well. (Busfield, 1986)

Granville (1877) remarked that familiar association with one's inferiors was pernicious and therefore to be avoided. Many superintendents ran their asylums far away from the wards or even from the hospital premises, preferring to delegate their duties to junior colleagues. Certainly, they did not expect to be much in the company of patients.

It was, therefore, the attendants who were the front-line carers. They spent most of their time with the patients and learnt their skills from practical experience of working with mentally ill people. As the asylum system became firmly established, the attendants were, over the years, building up a fund of knowledge about caring for psychiatric patients which was often passed from one generation to the next as children followed their parents into asylum work. It was not until the 1890s, however, that a national scheme for training attendants recognized that there were skills and insights amongst this group of carers which could be drawn out and developed to the increased prestige of the asylums, of psychiatry and of doctors, and also to the improvement of the condition of patients.

REFERENCES

Abel-Smith, B. (1977) *A History of the Nursing Profession*, Heinemann, London.

Armstrong, D. (1983) *Political Anatomy of the Body*, Cambridge University Press, Cambridge.

Baldwin, J. A. (1971) *The Mental Hospital Services in the Psychiatric Service*, Oxford University Press, London, p. 45.

Busfield, J. (1986) *Managing Madness*, Hutchinson, London, pp. 261–2.

Carpenter, M. (1980) Asylum nursing before 1914; the history of labour, in *Rewriting Nursing History* (ed. C. Davies), Croom Helm, London.

Connolly, J. (1847) *The Construction and Government of Lunatic Asylums and Hospitals for the Insane*, John Churchill, London.

Cullen, W. (1780) *First Lines in the Practice of Physic*, Vol. 11, Elliot, Edinburgh, pp. 312–13.

Engels, F. (1969) *The Conditions of the Working Class in England*, Panther Books, London, p. 52.

Finnane, M. (1991) Irish psychiatry. Part 1: the formation of a profession, in *150 Years of British Psychiatry 1841–1991* (eds G. E. Berrios and H. Freeman), Gaskell, London.

Goldstein, J. (1984) *Professions and the French State*, University of Pennsylvania Press, Pennsylvania.

Granville, J. M. (1877) *The Care and Cure of the Insane*, Hardwicke and Bogue, London.

Hadwin, S. (1985) Quoted in *The Anatomy of Madness*, Vol. 1 *People and Ideas* (eds W. F. Bynum, R. Porter and M. Shepherd), Tavistock, London.

Hunter, R. and Macalpine, I. (1974) *Psychiatry for the Poor*, Dawsons of Pall Mall.

Korman, N. and Glennerster, N. (1990) *Hospital Closure*, Open University Press, Milton Keynes.

Maudsley, H. (1879) *The Pathology of Mind*, Macmillan, London, p. 156.

Mitchell, J. (1984) *What is to be Done about Illness and Health?*, Penguin, London.

Mundy, J. (1861) Five cardinal questions on administrative psychiatry. *Journal of Mental Science*, **7**, 352.

Nightingale, F. (1863) *Notes on Hospitals*, 3rd edn, Longman, London, p. 49.

Parry-Jones, W. L. (1972) *The Trade in Lunacy*, Routledge & Kegan Paul, London.

Scull, A. (1982) *Museums of Madness*, Penguin Books, London, p. 36.

Smith, L. D. (1988) Behind closed doors: lunatic asylum keepers 1800–1860. *Social History of Medicine*, **1** (3), 301–27.

Tredgold, A. F. (1909) The feeble-minded, a social report. *Eugenics Review*, **1**, 97–104.

Tuke, H. (1884) On the mental conditions in hypnotism. *Journal of Mental Science*, **29**, 55.

Walk, A. (1961) The history of mental nursing. *Journal of Mental Science*, **107**, 1–17.

White, A. (1885) The nomad poor of London. *Contemporary Review*, **17**, 714–27.

4

Training for the attendants

4.1 INTRODUCTION

By the time of the 1845 Lunatics Act, there was already a thriving institutional culture within the asylums, and as new asylums were built, they took
on and further developed this culture. The asylums reflected Victorian society
in miniature in that they were non-democratic, paternalistic and class-con-
scious (Jones, 1991). Their culture was further based on the recognition that
the vast majority of their patients came from the ranks of the extremely poor
who required very little in the way of welfare provision to improve their
lot in life. Some superintendents saw the asylums primarily as a means of
distributing welfare; others took a sterner view and considered their institutions as character-reforming agencies with the principal agents of reform
being the attendants.

The mid–19th century saw the development of two major institutional
systems, the penal system based on prisons and the asylum system. Both
came into being at a time when the cost of erecting numerous large and
security-conscious buildings was low because land and labour were cheap. It
was also a time when the standard of living for the mass of the population was
very low. Chadwick's (1842) important Report on the Sanitary Conditions of
the Labouring Classes refers to damp and squalid hovels without light or
washing facilities, surrounded by piles of refuse and filthy, stinking gutters,
making the inhabitants worse off than wild animals. The Report considered
that those admitted to asylums were more fortunate than the inmates of
prisons and workhouses. Asylum inmates were fed and clothed, housed in
dry wards, looked after, and provided with medical treatment – far more than
most could have hoped for in their lives outside the walls of the institution.

4.2 THE WORK OF THE ATTENDANT

The attendants who looked after these patients with their varying afflictions
often arising from the exigencies of dire poverty led lives which were arduous
and akin to the lives of domestic servants. Their working day consisted of

cleaning, polishing and bed-making, dressing patients and serving their meals (Hunter and Macalpine, 1974). Supervision of patients at work on the farms, in the gardens and in the workshops formed a large part of their duties. Patients also had to be supervised while using the airing courts and participating in sports, and while attending dances and concerts. The attendants had to ensure that security was maintained at all times to prevent both escapes and suicide attempts.

Of the 75 patients who died at Colney Hatch Asylum in 1859, 36 had been bedridden, paralysed and helpless for months, totally dependent on the attendants:

> All these required, before their termination, the more or less lengthened use of the water bed, and great attention was paid to diet: beef-tea, arrowroot, jellies, wine and fruit being added to or substituted for the ordinary diet when, owing to paralysis of the muscles of the tongue and throat, the power of deglutition was greatly impaired. . . . In the performance of these duties, and the cautious and painful offices required by the sick, I can speak emphatically of the great care and patience of the numerous Ward Attendants. (Hunter and Macalpine, 1974, p.89)

The attendants also had to care for violent and 'boisterous' patients without the use of force. In the 1860s, great efforts were made to outlaw aggressive behaviour towards patients, and attendants who treated patients roughly were liable to instant dismissal (Hunter, 1956). Attendants therefore had to rely on their own skills in handling highly disturbed patients. The middle to late 19th century might be considered as the 'golden age' of mental nursing when the emphasis was on care because there was no other way of managing patients, and if patients got better, it was due to care. The impact of nursing could be less clearly seen when drugs and modern methods of physical treatment came to be introduced (Hunter, 1956).

The attendants administered such treatments as cold dressings and poultices, formentations, enemas and suppositories. They were also skilled in the technique of packing patients in wet sheets in order to control manic excitement (Urquhart, 1865). Baths of different kinds were very popular and given by the attendants. The Turkish bath was widely used and great and varied were the claims that were made on its behalf. Edgar Sheppard, Medical Superintendent at the Colney Hatch Asylum between 1862 and 1881, wrote in the Annual Report for 1866:

> These baths have remarkable powers . . . especially in Melancholia. . . . Sleep is wooed by its soft influence, and morbid fancies are chased away.

Other types of bath described in the same Report (1866) were 'hot baths for melancholia, cold for mania, plunge or prolonged, sat in or poured over, vapour or wet'. The Report, however, sounded a cautionary note on the need to observe better standards of hygiene. Not more than one patient at a time was to be placed in a bath, and the water was to be changed frequently; chamber-pots were forthwith not to be washed out in the baths!

The few drugs available at this time were prescribed and administered by the attendants on their own authority. Tobacco was used as a tranquillizer and, like beer and extra tea, snuff, sugar and cakes, were also given as a reward for good work. Sedatives such as alcohol, opium and hyoscine were used only sparingly as small allowances of dry tea and sugar could be used to placate violent or depressed patients 'especially if consumed at social functions such as tea parties on their wards' (Hunter and Macalpine, 1974).

Work was the major therapy in all asylums. Through work, it was considered that the mentally ill could be cured, rehabilitated and returned to the national labour pool. The attendants had above all to keep the patients properly employed:

> The great desideratum is to promote uninterrupted, interesting, varying employment, which strongly claims the attention, and leaves the morbid idea no time to develop itself. (Hunter and Macalpine, 1974, p. 127)

In 1852, over 100 occupations and trades were represented amongst the patients admitted to Colney Hatch Asylum. Whenever possible, patients were given work with which they were familiar. Apart from the loudly proclaimed therapeutic effects of work, it engaged patients away from the asylum premises, thus relieving the chronic overcrowding on the wards at least during the day. Patients who were good workers were highly valued and given the best food. There were instances where such patients were deliberately not discharged because of the income they generated for the hospital.

The attendants' hours of work were very long. Often the night shift undertook 'light work' during the day so that these staff worked from 10.00 a.m. with only a short break in the afternoon, until 2.00 a.m. the following morning (Quarterly Report of the West Riding Lunatic Asylum, 1880). In the 1880s, hours of work were slightly modified to include more off-duty time and some superintendents began to give thought to the comfort of their staff. Bevan Lewis of the West Riding Asylum ordered a reading and recreation room to be built in 1887 because:

> At present, after duty hours, if the weather be inclement or if the nurse does not desire to leave the building, she has no resource other than returning to her bedroom which in all cases is too small and too confined even as a sleeping room. (Mercier, 1894)

4.2.1 Duties of the Night Staff

In 1861, Dr Lockhart Robertson, Medical Superintendent at the Sussex Lunatic Asylum, published a paper arguing the advantages of employing regular night staff. Not only did they help to control the more boisterous patients, thus ensuring that the others had a peaceful night, but they also diminished the incidence of incontinence, thus reducing costs. Robertson considered that patients needed care 24 hours a day. His analysis of what the duties of night staff should consist of is illuminating (Robertson, 1861).

1. 8.00 p.m. – 10.00 p.m.
For the first two hours, the night attendants shall have the assistance of one of the day attendants by rotation.

2. 10.00 a.m. – 4.00 a.m.
Their first duty shall be to ascertain from the Head Attendant the names of patients requiring particular attention in the administering of medicine or other comforts for the sick, and of those disposed to acts of suicide. All such patients, as well as the epileptic patients, must be visited every hour during the watch.

3. The several wards shall be visited four times during the night, viz. at 10.00 p.m., midnight, 2.00 a.m. and 4.00 a.m. At each of these visits, all the epileptic patients and especially the paralytic shall be examined as to the state of the sheets; if these are soiled or wet they must be changed at once.

4. It is further the duty of the night attendants to become acquainted with the patients who habitually wet their beds, and all such patients must at each of the prescribed visits, if necessary, be awoke and called upon to attend to the calls of nature. With some patients, one such systematic call at midnight will suffice; with others it will be necessary to repeat the call at 2.00 a.m., while others require to be called four times during the night.

5. With the exception of epileptic patients in a fit, these precautions should entirely obviate all wet beds in the ordinary cases of chronic mental disease. It will also be found that enforced habits of cleanliness at night result in cleanly habits by day.

6. The night attendants will be careful to record in their night reports, each morning before going off duty, the number of patients visited and the number found wet and dirty.

4.2.2 Duties of the Head Attendant

The Head Attendant reported daily to the medical superintendent and it was through him that staff and patients made appointments to speak to the superintendent. He inspected all new patients and made an assessment of them to the doctor in charge. He was an important figure from the earliest days of the asylum system, although it was not until 1894 that Charles Mercier published the duties which had come to be associated with the post:

7.30 a.m	Breakfast
8.00 a.m.	Visit all wards
10.30 a.m.	Tour of inspection
1.30 p.m.	Dinner
2.00 p.m.	Supervise wards and airing courts
5.00 p.m.	Supervise patients' teas
10.00 p.m.	Masterlock all communication doors

These duties had been evolving since the birth of the asylum system and each Head Attendent would have formulated his own routines. By the mid-1890s, however, attempts were being made to regulate the work of asylum personnel on a national scale, both by publishing details of their duties as with Mercier's description above, and, more importantly, through the introduction of training schemes into the asylums.

4.2.3 Power of the Superintendents over the Attendants

The attendants were subject to the superintendent in every aspect of their working lives and large parts of their personal lives; two decades after the 1845 Act, the asylum system had become a paternalistic regime where the attendants were as much under the control of the superintendent as were the patients. At the West Riding Asylum, 91 out of 567 attendants were sacked by one superintendent during his reign of office for reasons varying from 'dishonesty to being found drunk' (Robertson, 1861). It is difficult to know whether such a dismissal rate was because this particular superintendent was drunk on his own power, or whether his ability to select suitable staff was poor, or whether the calibre of those who presented themselves for employment as attendants was so low that no amount of supervision could transform them into adequate nurses.

4.3 EARLY TRAINING OF THE ATTENDANTS

The limitations of the training for attendants were only equalled by the poverty of training available to doctors. Apart from the *Journal of Mental Science*, there were few opportunities for doctors to learn about the latest theories of mental illness and new treatments. Although certain individuals tried to improve the state of specialist psychiatric knowledge – Alexander Morrison,[1] an inspector of asylums, started in-house lectures for doctors at the Bethlem Hospital in 1823, John Connolly at the Hanwell Asylum in 1842, and Thomas Laycock in Edinburgh in the 1860s – it was not until

[1]Morrison (1779–1866) practised as a doctor and teacher in London and Edinburgh, and founded the Society for Improving the Conditions of the Insane in 1842. He sought to improve the care of mental patients by awarding prizes to doctors who wrote innovative essays dealing with aspects of patient care. He also awarded good conduct prizes to attendants.

1885 that the asylum doctors' own organization, the Medico-Psychological Association (MPA), persuaded the General Medical Council to introduce a Certificate in Psychological Medicine. Candidates had to have been resident in a hospital for 3 months and attended a course of lectures. Nobody applied for the first examination (Lewis, 1967).

Hunter (1956) argues that the training of attendants preceded that of doctors. He traces the origins of formal training back to the Retreat at York which was founded in 1796 on the moral management principle that:

> The influence of a healthy person's mind becomes the chief therapy in mental disease, and the mental nurse its most important agent. (Connolly, 1830)

It is doubtful, however, if Connolly provided any systematic training for his attendants. Simpson (1980) finds that the first organized course for attendants started at the Crichton Royal Hospital, Dumfries in 1851. Dr Browne advanced the course so that by 1854 it provided:

> A full, if popular, discussion of insanity in the different forms, intelligible by the shrewd and sensible, if somewhat illiterate class of persons employed as attendants and nurses. (Simpson, 1980)

From October 1854 to May 1855, Dr Browne gave a course of 30 lectures on mental diseases and their management to the medical and nursing staff at Crichton Royal. Thereafter superintendents in other institutions started short courses for their staff dealing with pathology, management and nursing (Abel-Smith, 1960).

As more training schemes were established, it became apparent that there was considerable variety in structure and content from institution to institution. The subject matter and style of teaching depended largely on the particular interests and abilities of the doctors who taught the courses. Nor were the doctors necessarily motivated by the desire to improve patient care. Carpenter (1980) argues that the medical profession was keen to take responsibility for the training of attendants mainly because it wanted to prevent any other group from so doing. Indeed, the first doctors to be involved in training had very little material of any scientific respectability to teach. It was not until they themselves began to receive proper training that training for the attendants truly got under way.

Training for the attendants was caught up and advanced by mid-19th century thinking and writing about the power of education as a tool of social transformation. John Stuart Mill called for compulsory education for all. Herbert Spencer and Thomas Huxley considered education a means of self-improvement, and of creating a disciplined work-force to service the new industries (Barnard, 1968). Various governments worked on the development of a national educational strategy and the culmination of their efforts came with the 1870 Education Act. This inaugurated a schools building programme and encouraged employers to contribute towards the establishment of 'Institutes' where their employees could take evening courses. The Act recognized that an educated and trained work-force would improve productivity and Britain's competitiveness in world markets. It was, therefore, entirely in keeping with what was happening politically and philosophically in the country at large when, in 1871, Henry Maudsley propounded to the asylum superintendents the advantages of educating nurses. He also asked the MPA to set up a register of 'good attendants' in order to improve their status and encourage high quality candidates to come forward for nursing work (Adams, 1969).

Further influences on attendant training came from across the Atlantic in the discourses offered to the MPA by Dr Kirkbride of the Pennsylvania Hospital. Dr Kirkbride was the driving force behind the founding of several psychiatric hospitals in the USA run on the principles of non-restraint. In 1843, he introduced a course of instruction for his attendants and became a tireless and well-travelled advocate of training. In 1882, Miss Richards, the Matron, and Dr Cowles, the Medical Superintendent at the McLean Asylum in Waverly, Massachussets, established the first purpose-built School of Nursing anywhere in the world. Here, formal training was provided for carers of the mentally ill (Church, 1987). Fifteen women graduated from the first class in 1886, and in the same year, the first men were admitted for training. (The School closed in 1968 when all specialized nurse education programmes were finally amalgamated into generalized nursing courses; Peplau, 1989.) In 1883, a second School of Nursing opened in Buffalo State Hospital in New York, and by 1899, there were 12 state hospitals in New York which had Schools of Nursing attached. Kirkbride reported these developments to the MPA along with his view that the training of nurses was an essential part of the medicalization of psychiatry.

Some doctors felt that training alone could not address the major difficulties of recruiting and retaining suitable people as attendants. The medical fraternity was also anxious that trained nurses might pose a threat to the power of doctors. What was happening in the USA in terms of the education of nurses was seen as so disturbing that Dr Cowles from the McLean Asylum had to reassure his colleagues at the MPA that:

> At the McLean Asylum, the nurses are not taught to write theses and the like; they are quietly handed their diplomas when they are due, and there is rigid avoidance of promoting any other spirit than that of aiming at modest, quiet, unobtrusive devotion to honest work. (Church, 1987)

By the beginning of the 1880s, there were still only a few training schemes of any consequence in this country. Interest was greatly increased when evidence began to appear that trained attendants had a demonstrable effect on the outcome of psychiatric illness. In his Presidential Address to the Association of Mental Science in 1884, Dr Rayner observed:

I have been so strongly impressed by the improvement occurring in the most unhopeful cases as a result of the bestowal of special care, that I have come to regard the one [training] as having a direct relation to the other. (Rayner, 1884)

4.4 THE HANDBOOK FOR ATTENDANTS ON THE INSANE

The MPA finally accepted that there was some advantage in training attendants and at a meeting of the Association in Glasgow on 21 February 1884, Drs Campbell Clark, McIvor Campbell, Turnbull and Urquart were commissioned to prepare a handbook which would help attendants 'to a due understanding of the work in which they were engaged' (Rollin, 1986). In 1885, they completed their task and *The Handbook for the Instruction of Attendants on the Insane* was published in the same year that Lord Shaftesbury, the architect of the asylum system, died. The first volume contained 64 pages, bound in red hardboard, with an appendix listing all the Public and Private Lunatic Asylums in the UK and their superintendents. So popular did the book prove to be that by 1902, 15 000 copies had been sold. The text was divided into chapters under the following headings:

1. The body: its general functions and disorders.
2. The nursing of the sick.
3. Mind and its disorders.
4. The care of the insane.
5. The general duties of attendants.

The Handbook proclaimed that the first duty of the attendant was to exercise personal discipline and to impose discipline on patients by setting an example of industry, order, cleanliness and obedience. The book summarized much of the content of courses then being offered to attendants. Many doctors regarded it as a significant advance in the progress of mental nursing because it represented a shift from the oral tradition through which the work of mental nurses had previously been described, to a written one. There were some, however, who viewed the Handbook with suspicion. One reviewer (unnamed) in the *Journal of Mental Science* questioned the desirability of offering such written material to attendants and wondered whether training could address the real problems confronting psychiatric practice:

We are not quite sure ourselves whether it is necessary or wise to attempt to convey instructions in physiology, etc., to ordinary attendants. Will they be the better equipped for their duties for being told that the brain consists of grey and white matter and cement substance? We hardly see what is to be gained by superficial knowledge of this kind. (1885/86, Vol. 31, p. 149)

Without doubt, the Handbook was, however, a milestone in the history of the education of mental nurses. Although it contained medical rather than nursing knowledge, it gave the work of the attendants a semblance of scientific credibility and the beginnings of a literature base. It signalled to the attendants that book-learning was now going to be important in nursing; indeed, the Handbook became central to training so that nurses who wished to advance had to be able to read and quote from it. It also enabled the nursing practices of hospitals throughout the country to be unified in a way that had never been achieved before. The MPA updated the contents periodically and in 1923, when the seventh edition was published, it was renamed *The Handbook for Mental Nurses*. To generations of nurses it was known as *The Red Handbook*, partly because of its red cover and partly to distinguish it from *The Black Book – Shepherd's Manual of First Aid*, which was the St John Ambulance Association's manual, also used in mental nurse training. In April 1964, the ninth edition of the Handbook appeared under the editorship of the late Brian Ackner, who enlisted specialists to write the different chapters. After the June 1978 edition, the Education Committee of the Royal College of Psychiatrists declared the book out of date and decided not to commission a further edition (Rollin, 1986). Not until the 1982 Syllabus was there another such comprehensive attempt to address the process of mental nursing, with the emphasis this time on the skills of the mental nurse as opposed to the Handbook's description of the work.

4.5 TRAINING AFTER PUBLICATION OF THE HANDBOOK

Dr Shuttleworth's 1886 lectures to the attendants at the Royal Albert Asylum in Lancaster discussed the principles of first aid as propounded by the St John Ambulance Association's scheme; Matron helped to supervise the practical work. Male and female attendants were taught in separate classes and charged 2 shillings and 1 s 6 d, respectively, for the courses. Each pupil was advised to purchase Shepherd's *Manual of First Aid*, price 1 shilling, and a demonstration triangular bandage, price 6 d (Shuttleworth, 1886). The classes proved so popular that it became necessary to ensure that some attendants remained on the wards in order to supervise the patients! The emphasis was on the type of emergencies that nurses encountered during their work, e.g. suffocation, drowning, burns and scalds. The course examination was conducted by Surgeon-Major Hutton, one of the St John's examiners, and of the 15 men and 19 women who took the examination, only one woman failed. The success of the course may be attributed to its immediate relevance to the daily work of the nurses.

Also in 1886, Dr Hitchcock of the York Asylum reported that not only were the attendants interested in the course he had organized, but many of the patients wanted to attend as well! Despite their enthusiasm, the doctor felt that this was inadvisable (Hitchcock, 1886). In response to the attendants' manifest eagerness for more knowledge, another book for them was published in 1886 entitled *Lectures on the Care and Treatment of the Insane, for the Instruction of Attendants and Nurses*. This was written by Dr Williamson, Medical Officer for the Insane at Paramatta, who wrote in his Introduction to the 70-page book:

> No mere book-reading will make a good attendant out of a bad one. Nevertheless, we believe that a few well-chosen practical directions will help to make a good attendant better. (Williamson, 1886)

His text dealt with four areas.

1. Obedience and discipline.
   Personal neatness and courtesy to patients.
   The avoidance of ridiculing delusions.
   The importance of comfort for all in the asylum.

2. Care and observation of epileptic patients.
   Care and observation of suicidal patients.
   Restraint, seclusion and artificial feeding.

3. Bandaging and treatment of wounds, sores, bruises and burns.
   Bathing patients.

4. Importance of occupation, amusements and religious services.

According to Williamson the role of the attendant was to carry out medical instructions, and to care for and supervise large numbers of patients. He found supervision to be often inadequate:

> Black eyes, cut faces, bruises and scalp wounds received by epileptics or by other patients in conflict with them are in a large number of instances evidence of a lack of proper supervision. (Williamson, 1886)

Strahan (1886) argued that the purpose of training went further than instructing attendants in how to care for patients. The attendants had also to be made aware of the broader medical context of psychiatry and the part they had to play in the service of psychiatry. Medicine, he argued, was potentiated by attendants familiar with the elementary principles of nursing.

Courses such as these which responded to a desire on the part of the attendants to learn and improve themselves combined with lobbying from various superintendents, finally convinced the MPA that a national training scheme was needed. Its 1889 Annual General Meeting unanimously approved the appointment of a special committee to report on such a scheme for asylum nurses and attendants. The committee was also to investigate the possibility of awarding a Certificate in Nursing the Insane and the registration of Certificate holders.

The committee worked rapidly to establish the requirements attendants must fulfil before sitting the MPA's examination. A 3 months probationary period had to be completed before attendants were accepted for training. Two years training and service in the asylum (which included the 3 months probationary period) had then to be undertaken. The Handbook was to be the basic training text, but other books could also be made available to attendants at the discretion of the superintendent. Lectures and demonstrations were to be given by the medical staff, although occasional practical exercises might be supervised by the Head Attendant. The superintendent would assess the trainees' progress by periodic tests.

Training aimed to give the attendants an understanding of bodily structure and function sufficient to qualify them to administer 'first aid', especially in relation to the type of accidents and injuries which occurred in the asylums. The syllabus concentrated on anatomy, physiology and first aid in the first year, and on physical and mental diseases and their management in the second. Although the training was modest by today's standards, the qualification was welcomed by the attendants and generally accepted as a passport to work in the private institutions, public asylums and the reformed Poor Law Infirmaries.

Examinations were held twice yearly in each asylum where there were candidates: on the first Monday in May and the first Monday in November. Candidates completed a schedule obtained from the Registrar and returned it with their examination fee of 2s 6d at least 4 weeks before the examination date. Resits were charged at the rate of 1 shilling. There was both a written paper and a viva voce. The questions were set by examiners appointed by the MPA, the same as examined medical students for the Association's Diploma. Written answers were marked by the superintendent and an outside assessor who was a superintendent from another asylum approved by the Association to act in this capacity. The practical part of the examination, which was held 2 or 3 days later, was conducted by the superintendent and the same external assessor.

No record of the first examination paper for attendants has been located to date, but the paper of the examination held in May 1893 was published in the *Journal of Mental Science*, and provides a fascinating insight into the type and degree of knowledge required of examinees (Table 4.1).

Similar questions appeared in subsequent exams and doubtless reflected those topics with which superintendents were most concerned their attendants should be familiar. The ability to detect abnormalities in specimens of urine was considered an important feature of the attendants' work (question 8), and their observations had to be conveyed to the superintendent through his daily meeting with the Head Attendant. It was medical opinion at this

Table 4.1 May 1893 examination for attendants on the insane

---

1. Mention the causes of lung disease.
2. By what channels is the refuse or waste matter of the body drained from the circulation?
3. What symptoms would lead you to suspect that a patient is losing weight?
4. What symptoms would lead you to suspect that a patient is gaining weight?
5. (a) What is a sensory nerve?
   (b) What is a motor nerve?
6. Name the special senses.
7. (a) What is a drawsheet?
   (b) Explain how you would use it.
   (c) What are its advantages?
8. (a) What observations would you make regarding the passing of urine and
   (b) the appearance of the urine?
9. (a) Why is occupation important in the treatment of the insane?
   (b) What rules should be observed in promoting the occupation of patients?
10. (a) What patients are most likely to escape?
    (b) What circumstances would make you suspicious?
    (c) How would you guard against escape?
11. (a) In what way should attendants conduct themselves towards patients?
    (b) What do you understand by 'showing a good example'?
12. (a) What are the risks in treating cases in private houses compared with asylums?
    (b) What precautions would you take?
13. What are the difficulties with relatives in private houses, and how would you endeavour to meet them?

---

time that occupation was not only a treatment for insanity but also provided a means by which patients' progress could be assessed. Those who were improving worked harder and those who were not manifested disinterest in their work (question 9). Some of the attendants who took the examination were working with patients in private madhouses or in their own homes, necessitating considerable diplomacy on their part in managing truculent behaviour under the eye of patients' relatives (question 13).

The results of both written and practical examinations had to be forwarded to the Registrar not later than 10 days from the date of the written examination. Once attendants' names were entered on the Association Register, their superintendents were held responsible for their conduct, and anyone found guilty of misconduct was to be reported to the Registrar who could remove his/her name from the Register and advise dismissal.

The first Registrar was Dr Beveridge Spence of the Burntwood Asylum, Lichfield; it was his job to co-ordinate and oversee the examinations and to keep a Register of those who passed. At the 1894 Annual Meeting of the Association, he reported that 29 institutions were preparing nurses for exami-

Table 4.2 Candidates prepared for the first examination, May 1891

Asylum	Male	Female
Birmingham Asylum	5	8
Rubery Asylum	2	4
James Murray's Royal Asylum, Perth	3	2
Kirklands Asylum, Bothwell	1	2
Stirling District Asylum, Larbert	4	4
Total	15	20

nation, and in October of that year, the Association decided that a badge should be issued to holders of its Certificate. This badge was not intended as a gift to the attendant, but was to remain the property of the asylum, and be returned with uniform, belt, keys and rule book at the termination of the attendant's employment. The badge was based on a cross pattern and the words 'For Proficiency in Mental Nursing' appeared on the arms of the cross. On a central disc was written 'Medico-Psychological Association' and there was a representation of Psyche with her butterfly wings.

The first list of those awarded the Association's 'Certificate of Proficiency in Nursing the Insane' was published in the *Journal of Mental Science* for October 1892. Only two English asylums, both in Birmingham, prepared candidates for the first examination, and the rest were in Scotland (Table 4.2).

In November 1891, eight asylums presented candidates and 31 males and 40 females were successful. By May 1892, 15 asylums were participating in the scheme and in the examination of that year, 70 males and 70 females were successful. Between May 1891 and May 1898, 1234 males and 1418 females were awarded Certificates. By 1899, over 100 asylums were participating in the training scheme and nearly 600 Certificates were being awarded each year. However, training remained confined almost entirely to the public asylums with only a few private institutions becoming involved. And despite the increase in the number of asylums providing training and in the number of trained personnel, dissatisfaction was simmering among mental nursing staff.

In the 1893 Annual Report of the Bethlem Hospital, it was remarked that training had contributed to a more hard-working and conscientious atmosphere among the 'servants' but that despite their keenness to attend lectures and demonstrations, few offered themselves for the examination. The Report stated ruefully that even senior staff could not be persuaded to face an examination, although they willingly attended lectures. It suggested that 'good candidates' who were likely to pass the examination should be entered initially in the hopes that their success would spur others on to attempt the papers.

4.6 THE ANTIPATHY OF MRS BEDFORD-FENWICK

Training for the attendants developed against a background of animosity from the leadership of the newly emerging group of qualified general nurses. Training for general nurses had started in 1860 at St Thomas's Hospital under the influence of Florence Nightingale. It was her intention that the nurses trained at St Thomas's should go out to train other nurses in the UK and in the rest of the world, using schemes based on the St Thomas's model. During the early 1880s, the increasing numbers of trained general nurses began to voice their dissatisfaction with a situation wherein training did not improve their career opportunities. Mrs Bedford-Fenwick, close associate of Florence Nightingale, wife of an M.P. and Matron of a large London hospital, together with a number of younger matrons, sought to link the cause of nursing with that of the women's suffragette movement. In 1887, Mrs Bedford-Fenwick founded the British Nursing Association (BNA) with the aim of acquiring a Royal Charter and state recognition for trained nurses. Princess Christian, a daughter of Queen Victoria, became the Association's first Patron. An executive council comprising both matrons and doctors was set up, and among the doctors were a number of prominent psychiatrists and neurologists, notably Sir James Crichton-Brown, Sir Dyce Duckworth and Dr Outterson-Wood (Adams, 1969).

Mental nursing did not feature in Florence Nightingale's grand plan, nor in Mrs Bedford-Fenwick's political agitations. In 1895, Sir Dyce Duckworth proposed to the now Royal British Nursing Association (RBNA) that those who passed the MPA's examination should be considered qualified to offer themselves for registration with the RBNA. The resolution was adopted in the absence of Mrs Fenwick who then wrote vigorously against it in the *Nursing Record*:

> Everyone will agree that no person can be considered trained who has only worked in hospitals and asylums for the insane. The proposal recommends that the register of trained nurses is open to men as well as to women and considering the present class of persons known as male attendants, one can hardly believe that their admission will tend to raise the status of the Association, while we foresee considerable trouble for the executive council from such members. (Bedford-Fenwick, 1896)

She also suggested in her Editorial that asylum workers could not be called nurses and that the MPAs training was inferior to that of general nurses. In conclusion, she urged all trained general nurses to protest strongly against Sir Dyce Duckworth's motion. Such was her influence that those who had supported the registration of asylum nurses were not invited to further meetings of the RBNA.

Nor were the attendants themselves at all happy about the motion which had been passed on their behalf. They were adamant that they did not want to be part of any Register which had been drawn up primarily for general nurses. Sir Dyce Duckworth's manoeuvrings, however, forced the attendants to recognize their need for an organization which would represent their own particular interests. There were members of the MPA who were not averse to this idea and who were prepared to facilitate the setting up of an 'Asylum Workers Association' (AWA) with the aim of promoting the interests and status of attendants and of others engaged in mental nursing. The doctors who supported the AWA saw it as beneficial to the respectability of psychiatry as a whole if the attendants of the mentally ill received greater recognition and were held in higher esteem. Well-respected nurses could but add to the prestige of the doctors who controlled them.

The medical fraternity thus went in two different directions in its efforts to improve the image of psychiatry and of the standing of its medical practitioners. Those of Sir Dyce Duckworth's party felt that the status of doctors would be better assured if mental nurses were to associate themselves with general nurses and so gain a vicarious respectability from them. The general nurses were after all well established now and basking in the eminence of Florence Nightingale. Other doctors preferred to see the attendants form their own Association separate from the general nurses, and thus remain a work-force exclusive to psychiatry and not subject to the influence of nurses working in different circumstances, who were more politically muscled than they and likely to make greater demands for pay, power and autonomy.

The AWA was mainly an organization for the attendants, although other asylum workers – maids, gardeners, stewards and tailors – also joined. The attendants feared any affiliation with general nurses and wanted to reinforce their separate identity because of their suspicion that general trained nurses might come to be employed in their stead in the asylums. The attendants felt that training had merely served to increase the prestige of asylum doctors and had offered them nothing. In their view, the medical profession had implemented training only to prefer ultimately the qualification of the general nurses.

The AWA published a monthly newssheet called *Asylum News* which aired topics of concern within the asylums and publicized social events, hospital teams, and theatrical productions. Much was written about pay and conditions, but little about training or the nature of the attendants' work. The newssheet did not attract a wide readership and membership of the Association was small in comparison to the number of attendants in employment nationally.

4.7 THE FAILURE OF TRAINING

In an extensive study of attendance in the West Midlands in the early part of the 19th century, Smith (1988) found that doctors had expectations of the attendants which they could not fulfil. Later in the century, the lunacy reformers and administrators realized that unsatisfactory nursing staff were adding to the problems in the asylums caused by severe overcrowding. Yet the introduction of training meant that staff who had been selected following the briefest of interviews and who had subsequently received what amounted to a very superficial training were expected to behave like well-educated, professional people. The MPA did not provide any ongoing training for the attendants after they had completed the basic training course. Neither did they invite the attendants to participate in the Association's meetings or facilitate the formation of any organization under the aegis of the MPA which would provide a forum for the attendants to discuss matters of concern to them.

Trained attendants were liable to public humiliation and serious penalties if they failed to satisfy their superintendents. Incidents of misconduct, which prior to the advent of the Register had been dealt with at local level, now became public. The first nurse to be reported for misconduct to the Council in 1892 was Lillian Ames who worked at the Fife and Kinross District Asylum, Cupar. Her superintendent, Dr Turnbull reported:

One of our nurses, Lillian Ames, passed the Attendants' Examination in May last and obtained the usual Certificate but has since been discharged from service here on account of becoming inefficient in her work and having behaved roughly to one of the patients. I . . . understand that such a circumstance ought to be reported to you in order that such notice of it may be taken on the Register as you may find necessary.[2]

Ames's name was not removed from the Register, but Fred Swadling, the next attendant to be reported for kicking a patient was given one month's notice at his asylum and removed from the Register. At the MPA's meeting of 21 November 1895, Emily Hartland's wrong-doings were exposed in a letter from Dr Woods, Superintendent of Hoxton House Asylum:

Emily Hartland was warned by me some weeks ago for encouraging two gentlemen resident here (one a patient and one a voluntary boarder) to make love to her . . . I am of the opinion that Emily Hartland is untrustworthy and immoral; unfit to have the care of asylum patients and to hold the Certificate of the Association.[3]

Christina Robertson's name was removed from the Register in 1897 after it

---

[2] At a meeting of the Council held on 17 November 1892 the Registrar read a letter from Dr , Turnbull detailing the incident in which Lillian Ames was involved. This letter is entered in the Register for Attendants held in the library of the Royal College of Psychiatrists.

[3] At a meeting of the Council held on 21 November 1895 a letter was read out by the Registrar from Dr Woods appertaining to Emily Hartland. This letter was entered in the Register for Attendants upon the Insane, held in the library of the Royal College of Psychiatrists.

was revealed that she had spent a short term in prison, and Joseph Lewis's name was removed for having deserted his wife to live with another woman.

These incidents reveal a very frail and vulnerable workforce of attendants – men and women of whom the highest Victorian standards were expected but who were, despite training, largely ignorant and down-trodden. It was unreasonable to demand professionalism from attendants who had no status, were underpaid, undervalued and overworked and whose training was superficial and controlled by practitioners working in a different field from them, namely medicine and not nursing.

Doctors did not see themselves as carers; their interest was in describing and classifying mental illnesses, and in the administration of the institutions. The responsibility of caring for the patients fell entirely to the attendants who often had:

> no higher conception of their office than that of a gaoler. (Annual Report of the Northern Borough Asylum, 1881)

Russell (1983) argues that doctors supported the introduction of training for attendants and claimed that training would correct shortcomings in care in order to distract attention from the more profound failure of the asylum system itself. The 'moral' treatment they had promised at the start of the asylum system had developed only into mindless routines by the late 19th century. It was much easier to point the finger at the inadequacies of the very human and ordinary nursing staff than to face up to the greater ineffectiveness that existed at the higher reaches of the lunacy profession:

> When the medical men found that the asylum system with its institutional pressure and its authoritarian structure could not be run without violent mishap, it was the nurses and attendants who carried the can. (Russell, 1983)

The medical profession found attendant training useful in bolstering its prestige. To have trained nurses on the wards enabled doctors to argue that caring for the insane was skilled work and so helped psychiatrists refute charges of inadequacy and amateurism. The truth was that psychiatry still had no scientific knowledge-base on which to ground its practice; nor were the attendants given anything of substance in terms of improved pay, conditions and career opportunities to render training a step in the direction of professionalization. It did not seem to the attendants that there was any difference in status between the untrained mental nurse and the trained, a situation which could but lead to low morale and falling standards of patient care.

REFERENCES

Abel-Smith, B. (1977) *A History of the Nursing Profession*, Heinemann, London.

Adams, F. R. (1969) From Association to Union – A professional organisation for attendants, 1869–1919. *British Journal of Psychiatry*, 20, 11–26.

Barnard, H. C. (1968) *A History of English Education*, University of London Press Ltd.

Bedford-Fenwick, E. (1896) On male attendants. *Nursing Record*, 2, 429.

Carpenter, M. (1985) *They Still Go Marching On – a celebration of COHSE's first 75 years*, COHSE Publication.

Chadwick, E. (1842) *Report on the Sanitary Conditions of the Labouring Population of Great Britain*, 1965 edition (ed. M. W. Flinn), Edinburgh University Press, Edinburgh.

Church, M. C. (1987) The emergence of training programmes for asylum nursing at the turn of the century, in *Nursing History: the state of the art* (ed. C. Maggs), Croom Helm, London, p. 76.

Connolly, J. (1830) *An Inquiry Concerning the Indications of Insanity with Suggestions for the Better Protection and Care of the Insane*, Taylor, London, p. 31.

Hitchcock, C. K. (1886) Asylum Reports for 1884. *Journal of Mental Science*, 32, p. 146.

Hunter, R. (1956) The rise and fall of mental nursing. *The Lancet*, 1, 14 January.

Hunter, R. and Macalpine, I. (1974) *Psychiatry for the Poor*, Dawsons of Pall Mall.

Jones, K. (1991) The culture of the mental hospital, in *150 Years of British Psychiatry 1841–1991* (eds. G. E. Berrios and H. Freeman), Gaskell, London.

Lewis, A. (1967) *The State of Psychiatry*, Routledge and Kegan Paul, London.

Mercier, C. (1894) *Lunatic Asylums: their organisation and management*, Lewis, London, p. 280.

Peplau, H. E. (1989) Future directions in psychiatric nursing from the perspectives of history. *ournal of Psychosocial Nursing*, 27, 18–28.

Rayner, H. (1884) Presidential Address to the Medico-Psychological Association. *Journal of Mental Science*, 30, 352.

Robertson, C. L. (1861) Some results of night nursing at the Sussex lunatic asylum. *Journal of Mental Science*, 7, 391–8.

Rollin, H. R. (1986) *The Red Handbook: an Historic Centenary*, Bulletin of the Royal College of Psychiatrists, Vol. 10, p. 279.

Russell, R. (1983) Mental physicians and their patients. Unpublished PhD thesis, University of Sheffield.

Shuttleworth, H. (1886) St. John ambulance classes for asylum attendants. *Journal of Mental Science*, 32, 200.

Simpson, R. (1980) Psychiatric nursing – what now? *Nursing Times*, 76, 10–20.

Smith, L. D. (1988) Behind closed doors: lunatic asylum keepers 1800–1860. *Social History of Medicine*, 1, 301–27.

Strahan, S. A. K. (1886) Can the medical spirit be kept up in asylums for the insane? *Journal of Mental Science*, 32, 349.

Urquhart, D. (1865) *Manual of the Turkish Bath*, Library of the Royal College of Psychiatrists.

Williamson, M. (1886) *Lectures on the Care and Treatment of the Insane, for the Instruction of Attendants and Nurses*. Privately published.

5

Mental nursing in the early 20th century

5.1 WORKING CONDITIONS

Life at the end of the 19th century in private lunatic asylums in the East Riding of Yorkshire is described by Russell (1983):

> The smallest asylums aimed at a homely atmosphere, where the patients dined with the owner and his family, where daily prayers were read, the Parish Church attended and country walks taken.

The same author considers the situation in the public asylums to have been very different:

> It is ironic that the erection of the enormous Victorian public asylums, like the one built at Willerby in 1884, made the lot of the confined mentally ill infinitely worse than it had been under private enterprise.

Nor did the introduction of training for attendants, it seems, bring about the transformation in patient care that some had hoped for. The old problems of increasing numbers of patients and difficulty in retaining staff continued to thwart efforts to improve the quality of institutional care. At the Old Manor Asylum in Salisbury, the superintendent sought to stamp out what he considered 'lax practices' on the part of the attendants and nurses by introducing amendments to the Rule Book. His revisions reveal both his own concern for discipline and agitation by the attendants for better working conditions:

General rules
1. Before leaving the employ of the asylum, one month's notice to be given in writing.
2. Instant discharge for disobedience, intoxication, absence without leave, quarrels, bad language, cruelty or neglect of patients.
3. Attendants to rise at 6.00 a.m. March–October and at 6.30 a.m. October–March.
   Attendants to retire at 10.00 p.m.

4. Men – Hair cut once a month.
 – Clean linen twice weekly.
5. Rules for leave
   (a) One day off per month: 7.00 a.m. – 9.30 p.m.
   (b) Leave every third Sunday: 1.00 p.m. – 9.30 p.m.
   (c) One evening off per week.
   (d) Married attendants – one night off per month.
   (e) Fourteen days annual leave after one year's service.

The 45th Annual Report of the General Board of Commissioners in Lunacy for Scotland (1907) emphasized the difficulty of staffing the institutions, a situation reflected in England. The Report showed that in 1902, 2056 staff left the service and that 1151 of these were dismissed for misconduct. By 1906, the numbers leaving had increased to 2292, 1248 of whom were dismissed for misconduct. Wastage rates had therefore increased in the 4-year period from 74% to 76%. The Report summed up the situation as critical and called for an immediate public enquiry to focus on the main issues which were the following.

1. A totally unacceptable turnover of staff in the asylums.
2. An urgent need to attract high class attendants.
3. A need to attract married attendants.
4. Provision of better accommodation for all staff.
5. Over-rigid discipline requiring relaxation.
6. Improvement of working conditions, rates of pay and pension rights so as to bring these in line with the Prison Service.

The Report further recommended that Scottish asylum workers could improve patient care and their own conditions of work if they organized themselves along the lines of their English counterparts. In England, an association had been formed for Asylum Officers which included administrators, some doctors, Head Attendants, Matrons and those in charge of wards. The asylum workers were catered for by an association whose members were attendants, nurses, farm labourers, gardeners, bakers, cooks and housekeepers. These two groupings had separate negotiating bodies. The Scottish authorities failed to take into account, however, that despite such representation, conditions in English mental institutions, and staff morale, were very poor.

5.2 THE NATIONAL ASYLUM WORKER'S UNION

The passing of the Asylum Officer's Superannuation Act in 1909 sparked off a series of confrontations between attendants and management. The Act provided for superannuation to be deducted at source from the attendants' wages. This was much less generous than the schemes hitherto adopted by many authorities under the provisions of the Lunacy Act 1890. Formerly, staff had often not had to contribute towards their superannuation at all; in Lancashire, for example, attendants had their superannuation paid for by their employing authority under the 'Lancashire Pensions Scheme'. As one would expect, attendants employed within this scheme were resistant to the new Act's arrangements.

The attendants found it difficult to organize, however, as superintendents had always fiercely opposed their attempts to unionize, dismissing those who were politically active in any way. Where staff did group together, the term 'Association' was preferred as less inflammatory than 'Union'. Nor were asylum staff allowed to meet to discuss their work and conditions within the asylums; they had to find outside venues. At such meetings, there was heated discussion about working conditions which were generally agreed to be atrocious. The majority of attendants were working a 90-hour week. The average pay for a male probationer was £26 per annum and for a female, £18 per annum. The result of all this was that in 1910, only 36% of staff in Lancashire asylums had given over 5 years service.

At the Mason's Arms Hotel in Manchester on 9 July 1910, a resolution was carried that a Union (the name was deliberately chosen to be provocative) be established for mental hospital workers. A second meeting was held at the Boar's Head Hotel in Preston on 24 September 1910. It was here that the new Union was christened 'The National Asylum Workers' Union' (NAWU). Whereas the 'Asylum Workers' Association' had come into existence under the partial aegis of the Medico-Psychological Association (MPA), the NAWU was the creation of the attendants alone. Mr E. Edmondson was appointed Chairman and Mr Geo. Gibson, Secretary, and there were representatives from mental hospitals at Prestwich, Rainhill, Whittingham, Lancaster and Winwick. Fuelled by the resentment aroused by the Superannuation Act, membership of the NAWU grew rapidly. The tone of its meetings reflected a distrust of management and the fear of exploitation. Superintendents refused to meet representatives of the Union or to enter into any discussion on the issues which were of concern to attendants.

The Union put its first series of demands to the Asylum Board on 7 January 1918.

1. A permanent advance on wages of 5 shillings per week for all staff.
2. Payment of wages weekly.
3. An increase of 0.5 d an hour for all artisans, labourers and stokers.
4. A 60-hour week with overtime paid at the rate of time and a half.
5. The practice of retaining a month's wages in hand to be discontinued.
6. 1 s 6 d per night for married men compelled to sleep in institutions.
7. An award of £2. 10 s on passing the Medico-Psychological Association's examination.
8. Permission to post Union notices in the institutions' mess rooms.

9.   Dietary lists to be posted in the mess rooms weekly.

The Board responded on 3 June; it granted the attendants the 5 shillings advance, and refused all their other requests. Relations between attendants and management became increasingly fraught thereafter, and came to a head in the first strike in the history of the English asylum service. This took place on 4th and 5th September 1918; at Prestwich Asylum, 200 staff were involved, at Whittington, 429, and at Winwick, a small number of attendants stopped work for a brief period on both days.

The following month, a 5-day strike was held at Bodmin Asylum where female employees tried to draw attention to their long hours of duty, bad working conditions and the systematic petty tyranny to which they were subjected. The nurses wore their Union badges openly whilst on duty, result-ing in the superintendant's dismissing 50 members of staff. A Visiting Com-mittee urgently arranged by the Asylum Board heard evidence from the superintendent and staff and subsequently passed the following resolution:

> The Visiting Committee recognizes the NAWU and that the asylum employees, being members of the Union, should be allowed to wear the official badge in such a position as not to cause injury to patients. The Committee has decided, solely in the interests of the patients, to reinstate all the attendants on strike.

Encouraged by this positive outcome from the 'Bodmin incident', the Union became more assertive in its demands for better conditions, and throughout the early part of the 1920s, there were a number of disputes. In December 1920, there was a strike (stay-in) at Cheadle Asylum; in September of the same year, a strike took place at Lincoln Asylum, and in April, 1922, another at the Nottinghamshire County Mental Hospital. This last was particularly volatile as staff and patients joined forces to fight police sent to restore order. The circumstances surrounding the death of a patient at the Salop Mental Hospital in February 1923 gave rise to an enquiry into conditions there. Both the working environment and nursing practices were found to be grossly substandard.

On the evening of 8 February 1921, the Rev. Gordon Lang, prospective Labour candidate for Monmouth, addressed a meeting of the NAWU at the Red Lion Hotel in Gloucester. He told his audience that mental nurses had a duty to demand better pay and conditions because the welfare of patients depended upon their being cared for by contented and well-paid nurses. Any attempt, he argued, to cut wages should be earnestly resisted. Later that year, some concessions were made to attendants and nurses at Coney Hill Asylum near Gloucester. A staff club was opened in the hospital grounds where drinks could be obtained at a discount; a Christmas dance was arranged, and male staff were permitted time off on certain Saturdays to watch football matches!

In March 1923, there was an enquiry at Hull Asylum following complaints from women staff about conditions on the female wing of the institution. The staff pointed to the overcrowding of bathrooms where several patients were bathed in the same water; the lack of respect for patients' privacy; the dirty conditions of the lavatories; dirty kitchens; and the confinement of patients to dungeons for long periods. The enquiry endorsed these allegations, vindicated the staff and recommended a number of improvements. The NAWU took the credit for having made public the conditions in which nurses were working and patients being treated. Moving on from local disputes, the Union next tried to influence the Government more directly. Their efforts were rewarded when Mr Neville Chamberlain agreed to meet its delegation on 8 May 1923. On behalf of the Union, Mr Gibson presented the following agenda:

Improvement in the quality of training.
Reduction in hours of duty.
Reduction in the rapid turnover of staff.
Salaries to be on the same scale as for similar work outside the institutions.
Protection of staff exposed to infectious diseases.
Review of anomalies in the Asylum Officers Superannuation Act.

The Assistant Secretary of the Union condemned the policy of secrecy associated with mental hospitals and urged the appointment of a Royal Commission to enquire into their administration.

This meeting with a government minister was vitally important to nurses in boosting their confidence to speak publicly for themselves and their patients. Their new sense of being valued resulted in the formation in 1923 of the 'Mental Hospital Matrons' Association' which immediately declared its intention of collaborating with the NAWU. Both organizations recognized the primary importance of training in improving patient care and working conditions. The NAWU ceased to exist in 1931 having made a considerable contribution to identifying weaknesses within the asylum system and attempting to resolve them. Most importantly, it represented the start of nurses taking responsibility for directing their own destiny in the face of the power of the medical profession.

5.3 PSYCHIATRY IN THE 1920s

During the 1920s, Britain was recovering from the effects of a war unparalleled in its human and economic costs. The large numbers of soldiers returning from the battlegrounds found that the 'land fit for heroes' for which they had fought could not provide them with even the most ill-paid work. Taylor (1963) has identified those factors which, in addition to the massive financial and human expenditure of the First World War, contributed to Britain's economic decline; these were growth in population, the inability of British industry to compete in world markets, and a continuing policy of investing in the Empire rather than the mother country. Unemployment, an intractable problem during the 1920s, reached 2½ million in 1930 out of a total population of 39 million. Unemployment benefits remained inadequate to meet even the basic needs of the unemployed and their families. Anger and frustration vented themselves in numerous small-scale strikes culminating in the General Strike of 1926. Ex-soldiers were particularly bitter, feeling that they had been neglected after serving their country during the War. The plight of the poor was exacerbated by the fact that those in secure work were better off economically than they had ever been before, resulting in a country uneasily divided into the 'haves' and the 'have nots'.

From the mid-19th century, there was a steady increase in admissions to mental hospitals. In 1890, there had been 86 067 people detained under the lunacy laws; by 1920 that number had increased to 120 344, and in 1930, there were an estimated 142 000 mental patients in hospitals in Britain (Ramon, 1985). During the early part of the 1920s, large numbers of soldiers were admitted suffering from shell-shock which was described as a functional nervous disorder requiring treatment by psychiatrists. Psychiatrists were then inclining to the belief that most mental disorders were caused by disturbances in the nerves or in the brain (Newton, 1988), this view slowly replacing the earlier 'moral' outlook which had seen the therapeutic potential of hospitals as centring on their capacity to regulate and reform the character of their inmates. British psychiatrists interested in the work of Adolf Meyer, a Swiss psychiatrist active in the USA for 30 years from 1892, attempted to reconcile the conflicting theories of organic psychiatry and of moral treatment in their approach to shell-shocked soldiers. Affected soldiers were immediately removed from the Front, and in hospital the men were offered group therapy and suggestion under hypnosis before being returned to active service as soon as possible.

This regimen was considered very successful, but while the War provided psychiatry with the opportunity to enhance its status, morale in mental hospitals fell very low. At the beginning of the War, many male nurses were called up for service, leaving the hospitals understaffed, and as the War progressed, the number of admissions increased, thus exacerbating the under-staffing situation. The cut-backs enforced by the Treasury on mental hospitals from 1914 to 1918 also took their toll on morale.

On 25 May 1919 the Ministry of Health came into existence and assumed control of the mental hospitals in place of the Home Office. The mental hospitals' Board of Control saw this transfer as signifying that psychiatry had finally been accepted as a branch of medicine with its own role to play in public health. Nonetheless, the Board was still very aware that the stigma associated with lunacy was an obstacle to the advancement of psychiatry and to the aftercare of patients.

Psychiatry was now beginning to recognize that patients came from the community and would have to return to it, but that the attitudes of society prevented rehabilitation of patients from becoming a reality. In response to this more socially orientated thinking, the Tavistock Clinic was opened in 1920 by a group of doctors who espoused the work of Freud. They rejected the institutional basis on which psychiatry had been founded and assumed that many people with psychiatric symptoms could be treated within the community. The Clinic was well received by the general public and was able to confirm that many patients with minor behavioural and emotional problems had, in the past, been too readily hospitalized. The Tavistock Clinic demonstrated that a limited amount of intervention and support could keep people out of hospital. For the first time, it was recognized that psychology had an important part to play in the development of the new model of psychiatry and should be one of the services it was now offering.

In 1924, the first psychiatric teaching hospital in Britain, the Maudsley, was opened. The Mental Hygiene Movement also took root at this time with the primary objective of preventing mental illness. It advocated a programme of prevention which would start with the unborn child and good antenatal care. Pregnant women were to be advised about their diet, taking exercises and avoiding infection. This was to be followed by regular physical and psychological checks on their children and early referral for signs of mental disorder. The first Child Guidance Clinic in England opened in London in 1927 and was from the start, run on multidisciplinary lines. The staff included a psychiatrist, an educational psychologist and a social worker. Their task was to deal with juvenile delinquency and other kinds of difficult and neurotic behaviour in children in the hopes that timely guidance would prevent more serious mental disturbances in adult life. This initial focus on paediatric psychiatric conditions gradually broadened to include liaison work with schools.

During the 1920s, as psychiatry gained in stature – the MPA became the Royal Medico-Psychological Association in 1926 – efforts were made to strengthen the body of psychiatric knowledge. Craig and Beaton's *Psychological Medicine* reached its fourth edition in 1926; much of the text dealt with the classification and symptomatology of mental disorders. In 1927, some of Freud's work appeared in Henderson and Gillespie's *A Textbook of Psychiatry*. This book presented the mental patient as 'a clinical abstract, without the slightest hint of a subjective dimension' (Ramon, 1985). Psychiatry was also employing new terms: 'hospital' was being preferred to 'asylum', and 'mental illness' and 'psychiatrist' to 'insanity' and 'asylum doctor'. The term 'nurse' now began to be used for both male and female carers.

In summarizing the beliefs underpinning the practice of psychiatry during the 1920s, Ramon (1985) finds that practitioners held psychiatry to be a scientific activity just as general medicine was; they considered the language of psychiatry to be objective and free from bias. Mental patients were categorized as unhealthy, low achievers, lacking in drive. They were both the victims of a faulty heredity and had brought mental illness upon themselves through their own irresponsibility. It was the task of psychiatrists to act on behalf of society to control the fertility of the mentally disordered and the essence of intervention was to provide a refuge for patients from everyday life through hospitalization.

5.4 MENTAL NURSING QUALIFICATIONS IN THE 1920s

The changes happening in psychiatry during the early 1920s found no parallel in mental nursing; indeed, mental nursing had made little progress in its practice since the end of the 19th century. The National Asylum Workers' Journal portrayed mental nurses as hard-working, dedicated, lowly paid men and women who identified strongly with working class culture. This self-congratulatory stance, however, was not echoed in the *Nursing Mirror* (1922) which thought mental nursing was in need of reform and should take general nursing as its model.

There were indeed moves afoot to bring mental nurses into line with other kinds of nurses. The Nurses' Registration Act for England, Scotland, Wales and Ireland received Royal assent at the end of 1919. This established a Register for general nurses with supplementary sections for other groups including mental nurses. It also authorized special uniforms for nurses and laid down the bounds of practice of registered nurses. There were to be penalties for the unauthorized use of the special uniforms and badges. At a meeting of the General Nursing Council (GNC) in May 1920, it was agreed to accept holders of the MPA's Certificate, and those holding the recently established Certificate for Nurses in Mental Subnormality, as eligible for admission to the supplementary Register.

In 1922, the first cohort of mental nurses trainees sat the GNC's recently introduced examination, which was very similar to that of the MPA. Of the 161 nurses who passed, 113 were female. The numbers of mental nurses registering with the GNC rose steadily until 1930 and thereafter, approximately 5000 nurses registered annually. Each year the number of females increased resulting in there being far more qualified female mental nurses than males. Not all who registered sat the GNC's exam as many who had taken the MPA's exam were entitled to be awarded the Registered Mental Nurse qualification on application to the GNC.

Mental nurse training in Britain still lagged far behind what was happening in the USA in the 1920s. There, psychiatric hospitals began to introduce postgraduate courses in nursing. Such was the enthusiasm for these courses that by 1929 there were 14 programmes running in 13 different states, varying in length from 2 to 6 months. The expansion of these courses soon exhausted the number of teachers capable of running them. This led to the setting up in 1943 of the first university-based teaching course for the preparation of teachers of psychiatric nursing. In 1920, Harriet Bailey published the first

American psychiatric nursing textbook entitled *Nursing Mental Disease*. The subject matter was disease-centres and directed nurses to focus on the somatic manifestations of illness, rather than on the whole person. It was not until the 1940s that a discernible shift away from nursing diseases to caring for people was evident in American psychiatric nursing (Peplau, 1989).

5.5 CONFESSIONS OF AN ASYLUM DOCTOR

Dr Montagu Lomax's *Confessions of an Asylum Doctor*, published in 1922, shook the world of psychiatry by the strength of its indictment of asylum practice. The book contained an account of Lomax's experience at Prestwich Asylum in Manchester. It was so unusual for a doctor to go on record criticizing his superiors that many sought to discredit his evidence on the grounds that he himself must be mentally disturbed. He described the asylum as gloomy, dilapidated and barrack-like, and the patients as poorly clad. Epileptics and tubercular patients were housed together and hygiene was negligible. The patients' diet was unappetizing; even when fresh meat and fish were included on the menu, untrained cooks failed to prepare it properly or present it attractively. Patients were drugged and purged and their lives were endlessly boring and dull.

The pay of Assistant Medical Officers, Lomax continued, was demoralizing in addition to their poor working and living conditions. He was unimpressed by asylum nurses whom he considered as lacking in tact, patience, sympathy and understanding, although even these failings were mild in comparison to those of some superintendents with whom he had worked. Lomax accused such men of neglecting their duties, of vanity, laziness, injustice, meanness and tyranny. Even if there were some committed and competent attendants, Lomax claimed that they could not be managed by such superintendents. The majority of superintendents considered that to subject the attendants to continuous supervision was all that was required for the smooth running of an institution. Supervision could compensate for the deficiencies of any work-force, no matter how bad their characters.

Some superintendents thought that training the attendants would eradicate faults of character. Lomax found this assumption to be mistaken. Training, as he had observed it, transmitted only knowledge and knowledge could not of itself produce a good character and good practice. Nurses, Lomax argued, had to be carefully selected, and the purpose of training was then to instruct these people, who were already compassionate by nature, in the delivery of a service which would effectively embody their compassion. Lomax sympathized with nurses in so far as he found their treatment generally, and particularly their rates of pay and hours of duty, a testament to the fact that psychiatry was far more interested in its public image than in supporting those closest to the patients. Nurses' working conditions were guaranteed to deter the kind of person needed in mental nursing from thinking of it as a career. The young unmarried nurses, male and female, led lives as drab as the patients' and they had no means of improving themselves. Lomax considered that when nurses were accused of low standards of care, this was because they were treating patients in the same way as they themselves were being treated.

Lomax's book probably did more to shake up psychiatry than all the meetings and edicts of the MPA. It resulted in a Royal Commission whose Report, published in 1923, was entitled 'Administration of Public Mental Hospitals' (Cmnd. 1730). The Commission found that many of Lomax's charges could not be substantiated or were exaggerated, but agreed with his overall conclusions that conditions for many mental patients were far from satisfactory, and that as long as such conditions prevailed, psychiatry stood little chance of being taken seriously as a branch of medicine. It recommended that forthwith, the size of mental hospitals should be limited to 1000 patients, and that superintendents should hold at least the Diploma in Psychological Medicine with experience as a House Surgeon or House Physician before their appointments. Patients were to be secluded only in certain clearly defined situations and were to be carefully monitored whilst in seclusion. The quality of food and the type of employment provided for patients was to be urgently reviewed, and aftercare facilities were to be developed in order to rehabilitate ex-patients. The Commission further urged Visiting Committees to be vigilant when carrying out their inspections. It considered that psychiatrists should develop a more scientific approach to their work so as to improve the effectiveness of their practice. As far as mental nursing was concerned, the Commission found it to be in great need of reform and directed it to base its practice on that of general nurses. In order to help achieve this, the Commissioners recommended that every mental hospital have at least one general nurse on its staff.

Lomax's book and simmering unrest in the mental hospitals also gave rise to another enquiry which was set up in 1922, the findings of which were published in 1924 under the title of 'Nursing in County and Borough Mental Hospitals'. This was the first ever official enquiry into mental nursing and was conducted independently of the MPA. As such, it was a document of the greatest significance. From the outset, the members of the enquiry recognized that mental nursing involved both the care of the chronically sick, and a wide variety of activities more difficult to define such as conversing with patients, motivating them, supervising them and participating in outdoor and indoor sports and work.

The Committee found that a concise definition embracing all the different facets of the mental nurse's work was impossible; instead, it formulated a set of principles around which mental nursing might develop.

1. In the treatment of mental disorders, skilled, tactful and kindly nursing is at least as essential as in the nursing of any other form of illness.
2. The standard of nursing required demands adequate training without

which it is undesirable that anyone be placed in charge of a ward for the mentally sick.

3. Training must involve systematic instruction, theoretical as well as practical, by qualified teachers.

4. Good training requires a wide variety of clinical experience, the realization of which for students may entail mutual co-operation between hospitals.

5. Governing authorities of mental hospitals must understand that considerable expenditure is required in order to provide a high quality training.

6. To prevent wastage, mental nursing should be regarded as a vocation and candidates for training should be bound by some form of contract.

7. As mentally ill patients are also liable to have bodily diseases, the nurses in attendance must have a knowledge of general nursing and that knowledge ought to be the foundation of their training. Conversely, the general nurse needs some acquaintance with elements of psychology and the practice of mental nursing.

8. It is fundamentally important to regard mental nursing not as a separate profession, but as a branch of the nursing profession. The ideal experience is that of complete training in both general and mental nursing.

It was somewhat paradoxical that, on the one hand, mental nursing was being directed towards the philosophies and practices of general nursing while on the other, it was being urged to recognize the uniqueness of its role in caring for the mentally ill. Unintentionally or otherwise, the Enquiry made clear its feeling that general nursing was the superior discipline by stating that mental nurses should ideally undertake both mental and general training, while general nurses need only spend a short time in mental nursing!

The Report did not take a stand on whether the GNC should have control of mental nursing, thus avoiding any dispute with either psychiatrists or mental nurses averse to such a move. On the whole, many psychiatrists welcomed the Report because they liked the element which linked mental nursing with general nursing, and thereby implied that psychiatric medicine was on a par with general medicine. They felt that any improvement in mental nursing could only serve to raise the overall standing of psychiatry. However, there were psychiatrists who did not relish the prospect of general nurse tutors taking over from them in the training of mental nurses, and this sentiment was widely shared by many mental nurses as well.

The Committee researched and presented for the first time data about mental hospitals and mental nurses in England (Tables 5.1 to 5.3) It found that the country had 97 hospitals with 108 646 beds. The largest of these was Whittingham Hospital near Preston with 2838 beds, and the smallest was Canterbury Hospital, now known as St Augustine's.

The evidence is clear that more women than men were employed as mental

Table 5.1 Average nurse:patient ratio

Daytime	1 nurse to 9 patients on male wards
	1 nurse to 10 patients on female wards
Night-time	1 nurse to 55 patients on male wards
	1 nurse to 56 patients on female wards

Table 5.2 Total number of posts nationally

Post	Male	Female
Chief male nurses	97	–
Matrons	–	97
Deputies/Assistants	93	110
Head nurses	86	149
Charges	1085	1300
Others	5187	6700
Night staff	870	1175
Total	7418	9531

Table 5.3 Number of nursing staff holding certificates

Rank	Male	Female
Charge nurses	510	635
Deputy charges	326	241
Day nurses	525	111
Night nurses	227	168
Total	1588	1155

nurses, but the total figure of 9531 includes a large number of 'others' who did not care directly for patients, such as ward domestics, cleaners, kitchen workers, and servants whose sole task it was to attend to the superintendent and his medical staff. The data do not reveal the high attrition rate in trained staff which meant that some hospitals had only three or four qualified staff in their employ, although the Committee did find that few staff had undertaken training: approximately one in seven of the men, and one in nine of the women. It was concerned that many staff holding senior positions had had no training whatsoever, and saw no benefit in undertaking it. It considered that the number of trained mental nurses was inadequate and that many employed as nurses were 'not the right type'. Those in control of mental nursing were asked to pay more attention to the selection and training of staff.

The Report recognized that merely recommending improvements without creating the conditions in which these improvements could take place was self-defeating. It therefore aimed to enhance the nurses' working environment, and the social facilities and academic opportunities available to them. It wanted hospitals to provide a nurses' infirmary and each nurse to have his or her own room and access to a bathroom, dining room and recreation room. The Report further suggested that nurses' homes should provide opportunities for developing *esprit de corps*, for making friends and for general enjoyment. It recommended the provision of extra-curricular activities such as hockey, croquet and swimming, and indoor recreation in the form of dances, concerts, whist drives and billiards.

As for training, the Report recommended that the initial period of tuition should be free from ward duties. Lecture rooms should be available and quiet rooms where nurses could study in private. There was also a need for refresher courses to keep nurses up to date. Teaching should take place in purpose-built Schools of Nursing, well equipped and suitable for fostering the corporate life of students. Ideally, these Schools should be separate from the hospitals, within their own gardens. They should also have an entrance which allowed visitors to be received without the necessity of introducing them into the hospital.

Despite the breadth and radical nature of these recommendations, the majority of mental nurses were entirely ignorant of the Report. In any case, the decline in the nation's economic state, and the underfunding of the psychiatric service made many of the recommendations impossible to implement. Nor did the Report address two major obstacles to improving the quality of care for mental patients: the social stigma attached to mental illness and the low pay awarded to nurses.

Although little action was taken following the 1924 Report, the Government remained eager to investigate the mental hospitals and set up another Royal Commission in July 1924, under the chairmanship of the Rt Hon. H. P. Macmillan. Its terms of reference were to enquire into the existing law and administrative machinery relaying to the certification, detention, and care of persons of unsound mind; and to consider the extent to which provision was or should be made for the treatment without certification of persons suffering from mental disorder. Much evidence was heard, some given by mental nurses.

The Commission noted with concern the wide variations in staffing levels throughout the country. It heard that in the refractory wards in Claybury Hospital, there was one nurse to 4.5 patients, while at the York Retreat, there was one nurse to less than two patients. At the Old Manor in Salisbury, a licenced madhouse, there was only 60 nurses to 672 patients.

The Commission also looked at the recruitment and training of nurses. It found that probationers were generally accepted at the age of 19 or 20 and that a large proportion left after only a short period. During 1924, 32% of women who left had not completed one year of service, marriage being the main cause of their attrition. Many entrants found mental nursing distasteful, while others were unable to conform to the rules or disliked training and sitting examinations. The Commission did not consider that to lower the age of entry into training would solve the national shortage of mental nurses; rather it recommended that hospitals should try and attract mature women between the ages of 27 and 35 years of age. To employ more women would help 'assimilate mental institutions to general hospitals', still considered a desirable goal.

Better technical training was called for and also that senior posts be filled by nurses who had undertaken both general and psychiatric training. Low standards of nursing care, the Report suggested, were partly due to the fact that two authorities were conducting examinations, the GNC and the Royal MPA. In the Report's opinion, this gave rise to conflicting loyalties and misunderstanding which were unnecessary as the syllabi were virtually identical.

The Report's emphasis on improved training did not find favour with many doctors who felt that the current training was already too advanced and unnecessarily wide in its scope for nurses. Dr Lomax, who was called to give evidence, found that nurse training was unduly difficult. Others believed that it was the demands of training that caused many nurses to leave, especially women:

> The book that the Medico-Psychological Association (has) put forward is far above the heads of the nurses to whom it is supplied. I would make it much simpler. . . . Really that book, as regards the nervous system, is one that I could very well put into the hands of gentlemen who are going in for the Diploma in Psychological Medicine. (Lomax, 1922)

The Commission's Chairman was sympathetic to this opinion:

> Personally, I would rather have nurses who were 90% kind than those who were 90% efficient in passing examinations.

5.6 REFLECTIONS OF MENTAL NURSES WHO TRAINED IN THE 1920s

The task of obtaining recollections from nurses who worked in mental hospitals during the 1920s was approached in two ways. The aim was to find nurses who, by virtue of having undertaken training, as well as having practised in mental nursing, could offer their impressions of both the practical and theoretical frameworks of psychiatric care. The starting point in obtaining a suitable sample was through the Retired Section of various hospital social clubs. These Sections included many individuals who could provide fascinating material regarding institutional life.

Adverts requesting potential respondents to contact the author were placed in local newspapers circulating within big cities. People who replied to the adverts were generally helpful in suggesting other likely candidates.

The sample eventually comprised eight men and four women who had worked as nurses in various mental hospitals in England during the 1920s.

More were interviewed, but their accounts discarded on the grounds that they could not be substantiated from other accessible sources. Some interviewees admitted that their reminiscences were unreliable due to illness, medication or memory disturbance.

The interview sought to elicit why the respondents had chosen to become mental nurses, of what their work had consisted, and their impressions of institutional life during the 1920s. Some of the interviewees felt they had been destined for nursing from the cradle. Their mothers and fathers had worked in hospitals which encouraged relatives of 'good staff' to apply for posts themselves. Other nurses had taken on the work as a 'stop gap' until something better came along, and others had simply been desperate for any kind of job.

One nurse gives this account of how he came to be employed as an attendant, a term used in his hospital until the end of the 1950s. Both his parents had worked at the asylum. They had met there, and he himself had grown up close to the hospital:

It never occurred to me that I would ever do anything else; it seemed inevitable. Ever since I was a small boy, I remember my father telling stories about what happened up at the asylum. He was Deputy-Head Attendant and it was his job to ensure that all the doors were securely locked each evening. On summer evenings, he used to take me with him and leave me in the Porters' Lodge while he did his rounds. I remember sitting in the big wooden chair with the Head Porter who was a kindly man and looking round at all the hooks on the wall with shiny bunches of keys and a whistle hanging from each of them.

He recalled two of the patients who came regularly to dig his father's garden; they had given him a little toy for his birthday. His mother used to give the patients tea and tobacco, welcoming them into her household so that her son never thought of them as odd or dangerous. So it was not surprising that when he joined the numbers of the hospital staff, he settled in quickly and found them 'a friendly bunch'. His first placement was on a 'colony ward' of 63 epileptic patients. There were periodic outbursts of violence to which some of the staff responded in kind, but the majority were compassionate and friendly towards the patients. He recalled one 'staff man' who would sit for hours in largely silent companionship with a young epileptic and help him compose a weekly letter to his mother who lived some distance away. These letters meant a great deal to her as she explained to the Charge Nurse:

The reason I keep coming to visit him despite the fact that he says so little to me is that I know from what he writes that he thinks the world of me, and deep down he loves me very much.

Another nurse who took up asylum work in the 1920s and who was eventually to become a Chief Male Nurse, recounts how he arrived at the asylum late on a winter's evening, and came in through a back entrance. (He had been instructed never to use the front entrance which was reserved for the superintendent and other such important people.) A porter in a splendid uniform greeted him and took some details before weighing him and directing him to the staff mess-room where he was given two pieces of bread and margarine and a piece of cheese. He was then taken to a small room leading off a ward where he got into one of the two beds and started reading:

> At about ten o'clock, the lights went out and some minutes later the door opened and an attendant came in obviously the worse for drink. I discovered later that on his day off every month he got drunk. He started swearing and shouting at me and told me to get the hell out of his bed. I was so scared I jumped out of bed and just as I was settling down, I heard him collapse on the floor. When I awoke in the morning, he was fast asleep on the floor and had obviously spent the night there.

Throughout the night, he was disturbed by the shouting and screaming of patients suffering with nightmares. In the morning, he was taken to an admission ward for 50 patients. There he was given a bucket, a bar of carbolic soap and a scrubbing brush and told to clean six side-rooms. The floors and walls were covered in excrement which was the result, so he was told, of the inmates having been dosed with large amounts of 'White Mixture'. Next he helped give the patients their breakfast which consisted of bread, margarine and porridge. He felt an outsider amongst the staff and did not find them friendly; later when they had got to know him, life became much better. His strongest impression of these early days was the frequent sound of bells and hooters:

> The day was punctuated by bells. The bell was rung at 6.30 a.m. to rise, 7.15 for breakfast, and at 8.35 for chapel at which every patient had to attend. At 10.00 a.m., another bell signalled that the working parties could pick up their packed lunches from the kitchen and go to work. At 12.45 p.m., a hooter sounded for dinner, the main meal of the day. The order and regularity resembled that of domestic service in country houses.

Some days after his arrival, he was taken onto the cricket field by the Head Attendant and put through his paces. Not meeting the required standard, he was never invited to play again. A few weeks later, he had a singing audition in the main hall at which he was more successful and the superintendent's wife, who was in charge of concerts, included him in rehearsals for the next pantomime.

One Irish girl, desperate for a job, had relatives working in an English mental hospital and having written to the superintendent, decided to take a job there because:

There was no chance of me getting a job in Ireland. I was so desperate that I was prepared to leave home and settle in another country. I thought at first I was going to do general nursing and when I discovered it was an asylum, I thought I would never be able to stick it. On arriving at the hospital, I told the Matron that I had helped in bringing up my younger sisters and brothers and had looked after my mother until her death. The Matron told me that was the best preparation for mental nursing.

The small number of those who came into mental nursing from Ireland had little education, but were willing to work hard and take orders. There were some Head Attendants and Matrons who were reluctant to employ Irish nurses because of a prejudice against them, but in rural hospitals where recruiting and retaining staff proved very difficult, they were welcomed. It often happened in such hospitals that Irish staff were asked to invite friends and relatives living in Ireland to come and work there. Many superintendents would visit Ireland simply for the purpose of recruiting nursing staff. It is still common today for Directors of Nursing to visit Ireland with a view to recruiting both trained and untrained nurses.

Another nurse told how he had joined the British Legion after returning from military service during the War. His prospects of finding even part-time work had been minimal. The Legion, however, was helping many ex-soldiers settle back into civilian life and secure employment and told him that there was plenty of work available at the local mental hospital where his recent army career would stand him in good stead. Accordingly, he had gone to the hospital, but had found it very difficult to get used to the work, and especially the attitude of the superintendent:

He had no time for me in particular and the staff in general; he regarded us as mere servants. . . . He was obsessed with cleanliness. He instructed us that hot water had to be used when scrubbing floors and steps, while the patients frequently had to bathe in cold water.

The nurse's life had deteriorated further when he became an activist within the Union and took it upon himself to inform the superintendent of how conditions could be improved for nurses and patients, comments which did not render the superintendent less suspicious of him!

I became the projectionist and was responsible for having the film ready each week. I used to have to travel ten miles to collect the new film and return the old one, taking in all half a day. A feature film was contained on four reels in four heavy cases. The superintendent, despite many protestations on my part, insisted that transportation of the films should be done on my half day off!

There was a small number of male staff who entered mental nursing direct

Table 5.4 The most appealing aspects of the work

Males	Females
1. Having a secure job	1. Caring for the patients
2. Amiable colleagues	2. Companionship of other nurses
3. Sporting facilities	3. Taking pride in the ward
4. Theatrical facilities	4. Walks with the patients
5. Indoor sporting facilities	5. Weekly staff dances

from Kneller Hall, the Military College of Music. Advertisements would appear in the College's Journal for competent musicians to become mental nurses. Hospital bandsmen were difficult to find and highly valued; these attendants often received special perks. They were entitled to extra food rations and also had more off-duty hours to allow for practising. On each occasion they played in public, they received a pay bonus. It was considered a great honour to be a member of the hospital band, because the skill of the musicians coupled with their sartorial splendour were an expression of the hospital's pride in itself. The hospital band also entertained staff and patients on special occasions such as staff dances, Christmas pantomimes, and at inter-hospital sporting events.

New staff undertook the most menial tasks and gradually advanced to slightly less unpleasant jobs as other newcomers arrived. Patients played a big part in helping new nurses to settle in, telling them what had to be done and how. For the most part, the new nurses learned the routines of airing-court duty, of farm work and of supervising football and cricket matches simply by observing what other staff did; there was very little formal guidance.

When asked to identify what they had most enjoyed about their work as mental nurses in the 1920s, male and female respondents differed in their replies (Table 5.4).

The women nurses tended to focus more on the actual work of mental nursing than on the perks, such as access to good sporting facilities. The ward and the 'family' of nursing colleagues fulfilled much of what they wanted from their jobs. Both men and women agreed that the least appealing aspects of their work were scrubbing floors and walls, general boredom, poor food and public reprimands.

The nurses felt that the superintendents were men who saw themselves as being socially and intellectually superior to all other nursing and medical staff in the asylum. They described them as careful to keep their distance, unwilling to establish any rapport with the nurses who, in their turn, considered them figures of uncompromising authority and conservatism. Superintendents enjoyed showing off 'their hospital' to visitors and only on these occasions would they try to give the impression that they were on familiar terms with the staff. The staff were expected to play their part on such visitations and draw a picture of their superintendents as great humanitarians:

Such social events were stage-managed and if staff did not comply, they would be severely reprimanded later. Conspiracy and deceit were practised widely, and as a young man, I had to learn quickly in order to survive.

On the 'ambulant wards', keeping patients 'quiet' was the main part of the nurses' work. These were the wards where staff complained of boredom, and where there was likely to be violence. Much time was spent in the airing courts. In one hospital, the wards would be emptied each day at 10.00 a.m. for an hour and a half, and after lunch for 3 hours, except in cold or wet weather when the afternoon session was reduced to 2 hours. Staff had either to stand at appointed places where they could best supervise what was going on, or constantly patrol.

There was no 'official' explanation as to why patients needed to spend such long periods in the airing courts. The staff provided their own reasons:

It was common to refer to the practice as 'airing the patients'. The superintendent often used to ask: 'Have the patients been aired?' It was widely believed that fresh air was good for people, particularly the sick and the mentally ill. The older staff used to tell us that bad smells and being cooped up inside drove people mad. I never heard anyone refer to it as a treatment, but it was frequently referred to as a good way of keeping patients occupied and out in the fresh air.

A staff-man who joined with me had previously worked at a big house as a footman. He told me that the high class family he had worked for regularly took long walks in the morning until lunch time. At least three times a week, he would drive them round the estate in a horse and trap in the afternoons. So there could be a link between what the top people did and what superintendents thought good for patients.

The superintendent at the hospital I worked at was Dr Thurnam who had spent a number of years at the Retreat, and his explanation for the importance of the airing court was that out in the open air, patients were closer to God. By that he meant they were close to nature and could witness the seasons change. He firmly believed it was nature that cured people.

The 'sick wards' were the home of patients who were either very ill or regarded as troublesome. Before breakfast, those who could shave themselves did so. There were only three or four razors to shave about 60 patients. When a patient had finished shaving, he handed the razor to the next and so on until all were shaved. Staff shaved the patients who could not manage for themselves, often using only two blades for 60 patients. The Charge Nurse carried the key to the razor cupboard and staff could not change the blades without his permission. Patients from the 'sick wards' were taken to the airing courts in their beds. Only the dying were left behind. On certain days, all patients were bathed, had their finger and toe nails clipped and were weighed. Each activity was recorded and the Head Attendant or the Matron then signed the record book in the presence of the superintendent.

One nurse reported that the most difficult placement he undertook during the 1920s was on an epileptic ward where staff tended to be 'rough and ready':

I remember the noise, shouting and aggression. Staff would get very short tempered and vent their frustration on the patients. Then patients would take reprisals and attack the staff member who had attacked them, and so it went on. Of course it was totally unhealthy to have so many people cooped up together in a confined space for such long periods. The staff were always looking forward to sports activities, presumably to get out in the fresh air and get rid of their frustration.

Those nurses who were training studied in their own time, learning from the 'Red Handbook' which each student had to purchase for him- or herself, price 1 s. 6 d. The training consisted of twice weekly one-hour lectures which started at 7.00 p.m. when the bulk of the day's work was finished. Practical lectures called 'demonstrations' were given on the wards by the Head Attendant, or if he was not a qualified first aider, by a representative of the St John's Ambulance Brigade. Fire drill was rehearsed and procedures explained for emergencies such as epileptic fits, apoplectic attacks, choking, haemorrhage and fights between patients. Surgical instruments were described, and information given on how they should be stored and cleaned. One nurse who trained in the 1920s describes the demonstrations he attended in 1924:

In my group, there were four probationers, two males and two females. We used to meet in a corner of one of the admission wards, close to a cupboard which contained surgical instruments. We stood throughout the lecture, and there were times when I nearly dropped off; we had been on duty since 6.30 a.m. We never knew what the topic was going to be until we got there. The teacher would give a demonstration after which each of us would have the opportunity to practice. The evening would end at exactly 8.00 p.m.

The theoretical lectures were given by doctors, mostly by the superintendents, and covered mental diseases. Epilepsy and dementia praecox (schizophrenia) received most attention. One nurse recalls how a doctor spent six consecutive weeks talking about the different types of fits. Devoting virtually all of the time allotted for training to these two conditions was reasonable because the majority of patients were diagnosed as suffering from one or the other.

Examinations were taken in three stages. At the end of one year was the

Preliminary Examination; after 18 months, the Intermediate, and at the end of 3 years came the Final. One nurse spoke of how:

> The exams meant a lot to us and we used to get quite serious about them. I don't remember anyone ever failing, though I do remember being told that, in the event of failure, we could take the exam again. The superintendent made it clear to us that if any of us failed, it would reflect badly on his training, and naturally we did not want to let him down. After we passed the Final, we were awarded £3.

5.7 CONCLUSION

The asylum system which had been founded in the mid-19th century was still flourishing in the 1920s and still recognizable as the Victorian creation it had originally been. The Victorian work ethos and mania for routine continued to prevail so that unless patients were very ill, they were expected to contribute through their labour to the upkeep of the hospital.

Staff were inducted into their work very quickly, becoming *au fait* with what was required of them within a few weeks. They cleaned, attended sick patients and supervised work parties. To stay busy and keep quiet were principles that applied equally to staff and patients. The routine of the airing courts remained a central feature of hospital life; it probably gave rise to more chronic boredom in staff and patients than it provided therapy for them. Training was largely irrelevant to nurses in the discharge of their duties, being based on medical theorizing rather than the actuality of the day to day situation on the wards. Staff were not close to patients and although there were instances of friendships between the two groups, the mental hospital was, for the most part, a place where patients found little consolation. Some of the female nurses apparently enjoyed making 'homes' on the wards, but the men were for the most part not greatly interested in patient care. They valued the job security which nursing offered them, and the perks such as sport and drama which the mental hospitals provided.

REFERENCES

Henderson, D. K. and Gillespie, R. D. (1927) *A Textbook of Psychiatry*, Oxford University Press, Oxford.

Lomax, M. (1922) *The Experiences of an Asylum Doctor*, George Allen & Unwin, London, p. 189.

Newton, J. (1988) *Preventing Mental Illness*, Routledge & Kegan Paul, London.

Peplau, H. E. (1980) Future directions in psychiatric nursing from the perspective of history. *Journal of Psychosocial Nursing*, **27**, 18–28.

Ramon, S. (1985) *Psychiatry in Britain – Meaning and Policy*, Croom Helm, London.

Russell (1983) *Mental Physicians and their Patients*, Unpublished PhD Thesis, Sheffield University.
Taylor, A. J. P. (1963) *The First World War*, Longman, London.

6

Mental nursing during the 1930s, 1940s and 1950s

6.1 INTRODUCTION

Asylums did not formally become hospitals until the introduction of the Mental Treatment Act in 1930. Although asylum doctors had long been talking about 'patients' with 'mental illness', and had constantly sought closer contact with general medicine, it was not until the passing of the Act that the concept of mental disorder as illness was cautiously accepted (Jones, 1991). This was the first major revision of mental health policy since the 1890 Lunacy Act and gave substance to such new ideas as observation wards, out-patient clinics and after-care facilities. It also provided for the voluntary admission of patients to mental hospitals. These imaginative and much needed reforms were not enthusiastically received by practitioners of psychiatry and the start of the Second World War did not create a favourable climate in which to implement them.

Throughout the 1920s and 1930s, psychiatric treatments had changed little, but there were signs that the cultural life of the hospitals was slowly beginning to abandon its military-style organization and embrace a more relaxed regime. Some of the impetus for this change can be attributed, remarkably enough, to the holiday camps which were becoming popular at this time. Sport took a greater part in mental hospital life than it had hitherto, and cricket and football teams were formed, comprising both staff and patients. Cricket players were provided with flannels, caps and blazers bearing the hospital crest, and the football team had its own distinctive 'strip' and would be followed by a coach load of enthusiastic supporters when playing away matches. Sports days were organized for staff, patients and relatives who joined together to enjoy an evening of singing and dancing afterwards (Jones, 1991).

The new legislation and the more relaxed style of such holiday-camp type activities did not mean that patients moved their position from the lowest rung of the hospital cultural ladder. Nonetheless, it was the patients who provided the labour which kept the whole enterprise of the asylum hospitals running and who adequately concealed whatever staff shortages there were.

Staff used patients as lackeys to carry out the menial tasks of everyday life, a relationship which did not help in the creation of a therapeutic environment.

During the 1930s, the position of medical superintendent of mental hospitals was a highly prestigious and authoritative one. Some superintendents attempted to overcome their isolation and the hierarchical nature of the hospital by communicating directly with staff and patients. Other superintendents were suspicious of such liberal attitudes; some never spoke to their staff, never entered the doctors' mess, had their food prepared separately and ate alone. Some even went so far as to have covered corridors erected between their houses and the hospital in order to eliminate any contact with staff or patients. The last Senior Medical Commissioner of the Board of Control, Dr Walter MacLay, was fully aware of the eccentricities of some of his colleagues and used to tell a joke about an admission certificate he had once seen. The certificate read:

This patient is arrogant, overbearing, and suffers from delusions of grandeur. He thinks he is a medical superintendent. In fact, he behaves just like a medical superintendent. (Jones, 1991)

6.2 THE WAR YEARS: OVERCROWDING AND COMMUNITY CARE

In August 1939, the Ministry of Health, in association with the Nuffield Provisional Hospital Trust, carried out a survey of hospitals in Britain. The purpose of the survey was to make available the 220 000 beds which it was estimated would be necessary for the casualties from the Second World War. The Ministry found there were 200 hospitals providing for the mentally ill and 150 institutions for the mentally handicapped. Most of these facilities were in the hands of local authorities, but subject to scrutiny by the Ministry of Health, the Home Office and the Board of Control. After the survey was presented to the Government, pressure was put on the mental hospitals to discharge patients and 140 000 patients from all types of hospitals including sanatoria were discharged (Titmus, 1950). Some commentators were cynical about this wholesale commandeering of beds from mental hospitals, seeing it as a reflection on the public's lack of interest in the mentally ill. Others argued that to release so many mental patients into the community bore witness to the Government's faith in psychiatry and its ability to cure mental disorder. Winston Churchill, however, was unenthusiastic about professional and institutional expansionism:

I am sure that it would be sensible to restrict as much as possible the work of these gentlemen (psychiatrists) who are capable of an immense amount of harm with what may easily degenerate into charlatanism. The tightest control should be kept over them, and they should not be allowed to gather themselves in large numbers upon the fighting services at the public's expense. There are, no doubt, easily recognisable cases which may benefit from treatment of this kind, but it is very wrong to disturb large numbers of healthy, normal men and women by asking the kind of questions in which psychiatrists specialise. There are quite enough hangers-on and camp followers already. (Churchill, 1951).

Some mental hospitals were completely emptied to make way for wounded soldiers and their patients were transferred to other hospitals which soon became severely overcrowded. From 1945 to 1959, the Ministry of Health's Annual Reports repeatedly highlighted shortage of beds, inadequate staffing levels and underfunding in Britain's mental hospitals (Webster, 1985). The founding of MIND in 1946 embodied the concern of some lay people about the welfare of mental patients. In June 1947, the Government responded to pressure from MIND when the Ministry of Health set up a Mental Health Division which was combined with the Board of Control. Local Authorities were ordered to appoint Mental Welfare Officers to take over the responsibilities of the Poor Law Officers. These Officers found that conditions in many hospitals were, in fact, worse than Ministry of Health Reports had indicated.

The population of the mental hospitals rose so sharply during the Second World War that it became imperative to relieve the pressure on them. Extramural services came to the fore and many hospitals began to establish rehabilitation wards and to set up therapeutic communities. Domiciliary visits and out-patient clinics were organized. At Warlingham Park Hospital, an open-door policy was initiated in 1951, partly to ease overcrowding and partly in recognition of the negative consequences of prolonged hospitalization, and the policy soon spread to other hospitals: Belmont in 1944, Mapperly in 1945, Dingleton in 1947 and Crichton Royal in 1950. The length of stay of mental patients became shorter and they were given more freedom within the hospitals (Ramon, 1985).

The shift of patient care to the community was based on three principles: firstly that it was better for the mentally ill to be in their own homes than in hospital; secondly, that community care was less expensive than hospitalization, and thirdly, that it involved no restraint upon the mentally ill. It was acknowledged that good care in the community required the whole-hearted co-operation of the local authorities, the public and social workers.

The haphazard nature of the mass discharge of patients during the late 1930s and early 1940s did not bear any relation to recovery rates. Psychiatry found itself travelling along two paths at this point in its history. Just as it was beginning to espouse a social model of care in the community, it was also pursuing with unequalled vigour new 'medical treatments' in the hospitals. Insulin therapy, ECT, psychosurgery and chemotherapy were in their heyday. While early discharge became common, readmission rates soared. This observation cast doubts on the long-term efficacy of the new treatments, but also suggested that local authorities did not have the resources to meet the increasing demands being put upon them by mental patients discharged into the community. Nor were GPs well informed about or, indeed, much interested in ex-psychiatric patients, their illnesses or their treatment (Goodwin, 1989).

The new treatments which were being tried out within the mental hospitals were being administered by staff who were very unsure about what they were doing. Clark (1964) comments that treatments in use during the Second World War and immediate post-War years had had little evaluation and that medical and nursing staff were ill-informed even about their supposed advantages, let alone possible hazards. Clinical staff had to live with ambiguity, claiming on the one hand to be engaged in treating curable illnesses, while on the other, feeling that many of their patients were suffering from psychoses of hereditary origin which would probably prevent their ever leaving hospital. The reality of care for such patients was not therapy but custody. Staff had to accept that custody involved strait-jackets, padded cells and forced feeding while projecting and trying to believe in their image as carers and healers. They adopted various strategies to hold these contradictions together:

> The most able and sensitive doctors either left the hospital and went into private practice or became the type of medical superintendent who interested himself in committee work, hospital administration or specialist topics such as forensic psychiatry. (Baruch and Treacher, 1978)

6.3 NURSING PRACTICE: TRADITIONAL AND INNOVATIVE

The 'Red Handbook' was still the basic text for mental nurse training during the 1940s. Some superintendents also recommended to their students texts which offered psychological explanations for mental illness, but which did not look at the care of patients. Articles on psychiatric nursing were available in the nursing press during the 1940s, but these were mostly written by doctors. In 1948, Fisher's *Modern Methods of Treatment – A Guide for Nurses* was published. This book saw the role of the nurse as primarily 'to be of assistance on the doctor'. Nurses implemented the treatment regimes of doctors, and kept the patients under observation so as to be able to report changes in their condition to the doctors. The book did consider, however, that nurses had the power to influence the well-being of patients:

> We all suffer more or less from mental disorder, but it is one of our greatest privileges in being alive that we can combat it in ourselves and others. That is why the joy of being a mental nurse is one of the best in the world. Even the probationer's simplest job of learning to make a bed properly and making a ward look nice represents the change from disorder,

and as she completes her training and her knowledge and responsibilities grow, the greatness of her work of healing develops. (Fisher, 1948)

Nurses were informed that the nature of mental illness was to plunge its victims into a sort of second childhood so that nursing became a question of washing, feeding and protecting patients from hurting themselves. The work of the nurse might seem unremarkable in the eyes of the outside world, but would be appreciated and remembered by those who benefitted from it. Nurses should not forget, however, that their care was insufficient without the strong right arm of treatment.

The book contained 10 chapters on treatments: sedation, relaxation, insulin and electro-convulsive therapies, pyretotherapy (malarial and sulphosin therapy), dietetic and vitamin therapy, endocrine and special drug therapies, operative intervention, rehabilitation and psychotherapy. The role of the nurse was defined in terms of her potential to assist with these treatments. Solely in the area of relaxation therapy might she have autonomy as a practitioner, employing natural methods of promoting relaxation such as breathing exercises, massage, or light therapy. The book considered massage as particularly helpful in inducing sleep, but warned that it was a technique which required many years of training to perfect. Relaxation exercises could be done in the bath in conjunction with hydrotherapy, and hot packs and sponging were considered to calm mildly disturbed patients. Jacobson's Progressive Relaxation was also highly thought of but in general, the book advised that relaxation therapy was suitable only for intelligent and co-operative patients!

The highly traditional image of mental nursing which Fisher's book conveyed did not, however, represent the whole truth about nursing practice during the War years. Innovations were afoot, and in some hospitals, nurses were assuming a more equal relationship with doctors and joining with them to move practice forward.

In the early 1940s, many nurses were called up, including some still in training, and assigned to the Royal Army Medical Corps. There they learned to handle medical emergencies and acquired psychotherapeutic skills which they would not have gained in training. Soldiers suffering from such conditions as neurasthenia were given priority admission to the Maudsley Hospital which soon became so overcrowded that new premises had to be found quickly. In 1940, a boarding school in the north of London was taken over and converted into the Mill Hill Emergency Military Hospital. Dr Maxwell Jones was in charge here and later at the Henderson Hospital in Sutton where many ex-prisoners of War returning from Japan were cared for. One of the first nurses to start training at Mill Hill in 1943 was Annie Altschul, later a Professor of Nursing. Her experiences there affected her profoundly:

The atmosphere at Mill Hill was refreshing after my general training which had consisted of lectures given by a tutor who treated everybody as if they were idiots. We had to suffer endless hours of dictation about things that bore no relevance to what I was interested in . . . But at Mill Hill, I found an excitement about the work that I had not encountered before. Everybody was expected to make a contribution. The staff, both doctors and nurses, were very keen to learn and every patient was regarded as interesting and someone from whom we could learn a lot. I worked with people I had only read about until then, Dr Maxwell Jones, Dr William Sargant and Dr Emanuel Miller and each of them made a considerable impression on me. (Altschul, 1991, personal communication)

Apart from three wards, two of which catered for uniformed civilians such as nurses, ambulancemen and fireman, and one for children, Mill Hill was essentially a military hospital staffed by health service employees. The military hierarchy managed it and the nurses had no duties other than caring. Every patient had an identified nurse who wrote up his report and discussed his progress with the doctors. There was an unwritten rule which stated that 'whatever patients did, staff should do too' and this meant that nurses were encouraged to broaden their horizons and take an interest in issues and activities beyond the hospital.

The morning shift was from 7.00 a.m. to 2.00 p.m., the afternoon from 1.00 p.m. to 9.00 p.m., and the night shift from 9.00 p.m. to 7.00 a.m. From 1.00 to 2.00 p.m., all staff met to hear a lecture from a consultant, a nurse or a visiting specialist. The lectures were:

Fascinating and most relevant to what we were doing. There was no training system as such, just interesting lectures. (Altschul, 1991, personal communication)

Staff were highly motivated to put the ideas they had heard discussed at these lectures into practice and as all had attended, all worked in harmony. The hospital provided an excellent learning environment under Maxwell Jones' influence. His aim was to make it both an educational community for the staff and a therapeutic community for the patients. The Assistant Matron, Miss Olive Griffiths, was equally inspired in her efforts to improve the quality of patient care and the education of her nurses. The importance of listening to patients in order to help them make sense of their experiences, and so as to understand and learn from them how to help other patients, was frequently stressed and generally practised.

Immediately after the war, Mill Hill was closed and the patients and nurses returned to the Maudsley. The nurses found the routines there antiquated and related more to the running of general than mental hospitals. Nonetheless, the training they had acquired at Mill Hill remained to influence them for the rest of their professional lives.

6.4 THE CASSEL HOSPITAL

A further contribution to the advancement of the mental nursing profession was made by the Cassel Hospital which had been founded by Sir Ernest Cassel in 1919. The hospital, especially under the Directorship of Dr Main, promoted the ongoing education of its staff, and, like Mill Hill, considered itself as providing both a therapeutic and a learning environment. Staff were encouraged to implement new approaches to care on the wards in the belief that constant evaluation and renewal of practice would provide patients with the best possible care.

In 1942, the founder's nephew established the Cassel Bursary Trust to fund research into the neuroses and care of patients suffering from them. Dr Main encouraged his nurses to take an academic interest in their work and at his instigation, the Trust funded a number of nurse beneficiaries. Elizabeth Barnes was seconded to the *Nursing Times* to study journalism and later became co-ordinator of an international study looking at psychological problems in general hospitals (Barnes, 1968). Gillian Elles, a tutor at the Cassel Hospital, investigated the cost of treating neurotic patients (Elles, 1968). Doreen Weddell studied the dilemma for nurses in being responsible both to doctors and to senior nurses and later became a member of the British Psycho-Analytical Society.

6.5 THE SOCIETY OF MENTAL NURSES

The hospital enquiries of the 1920s had considered mental nursing separately from general nursing, but those undertaken in the 1940s addressed the problems of both simultaneously. In 1943 the Rushcliffe Report appeared, more properly entitled 'The Report of the Nurses' Salaries Committee' which became a corner-stone for negotiations on pay and conditions and led to the setting up of the Nurses' and Midwives' Whitley Council in 1948. Endeavouring to improve the status of nursing and the quality of nurse training, the Report recommended that the working fortnight be reduced to 96 hours and that continuous night duty should not exceed 3 months for student nurses and 6 months for trained staff. It considered that all nurses should have 28 days holiday a year and one duty-free day per week, with sick pay graded according to length of service. For higher grades of staff, it decreed that salaries should be paid according to the number of beds in the hospital, a criterion that applied for the next 30 years.

Also in 1943, legislation in the form of a 'Nurses Act' was passed to try and tackle the chronic shortage of nursing staff. The Act created a new level of nurse who was Enrolled rather than Registered, and allowed 'bona fide' assistant nurses to apply to the General Nursing Council (GNC) for enrolment. This had the effect of substantially increasing the number of trained nurses at no extra cost. Despite this measure, it was still necessary to designate 'priority areas' that winter, so acute was the need for trained nurses in certain parts of the country.

Against this disparate background, 70 mental nurses met on 4th November 1943, under the aegis of the Royal College of Nursing's London Branch, to discuss organizational and educational matters appertaining to mental nursing. The recommendation of the Rushcliffe Committee that there should be national agreements on salaries and conditions of service effectively disenfranchized the mental nurses whose only voice was through the unions because they had no representation on the nurses' pay and conditions negotiating body. Disenchantment was widespread amongst mental nurses who felt uninvolved in schemes which would affect their future and their patients':

Mental nurses were doing good work under difficulties. Suggestions for improving their work could not be discussed with the nurses because there was no organisation through which they could be consulted. At that time the Royal College of Nursing admitted only general trained nurses. (Minutes of the Society of Mental Nurses, 1943)[1]

The meeting resulted in the setting up of the Society of Mental Nurses as a subgroup within the Royal College of Nursing (RCN). The instigators were female mental nurses who were members of the RCN by virtue of being additionally qualified as general nurses. It was agreed that the objectives of the Society were:

To promote the interests of mental nurses, to establish co-operation between them and other organisations of nurses, and to co-ordinate action upon matters affecting their interests . . . to promote and maintain such professional standards as will make constructive contribution to the nursing world and to the community.

Letters were read from nurses who wanted to become members of the new Society, but who were prevented from attending the first meeting by their medical superintendents. The Society was openly hostile to the power exercised by superintendents and although it had no statutory authority to represent mental nurses, its aim was to influence those who made decisions about mental nursing.

Not all present were of the opinion that a special interest group was the best way forward, even though they felt the need to bring the particular problems facing mental nurses to the fore. Some said that to start a new group specifically for mental nurses within the RCN would be to isolate themselves educationally and financially from mainstream nursing, and that it would be better to seek equality with general nurses within the College.

[1]This information was derived from *A Brief History of the Society of Mental Nurses, 1943–72* which is currently in the possession of Miss O. Griffith and about to be placed in the RCN Library, London.

The National Asylum Workers' Union was also opposed to the Society on the grounds that it would fragment representation of the mental nursing workforce.

The majority of nurses who joined the new Society still believed that mental nurses must remain united with colleagues from other branches of nursing or render themselves powerless. Several Matrons took exception to the General Nursing Council's placing mental nurses on a 'Supplementary Register' where 'supplementary', they felt, implied inferior. They wanted one Register to include both general and mental nurses, and argued that the exclusion of mental nurses from membership of the RCN should be revoked.

In 1948, the National Health Service came into being and psychiatry was absorbed into the new nationwide system of health care provision. In the same year, the last group of students to qualify under the Royal Medico-Psychological Association's scheme started their training; by 1951, training for mental nurses had passed entirely into the hands of the GNC. The Society of Mental Nurses preferred the GNC's training scheme on the grounds that it was far more thorough. It was certainly more like the general nurses' training programme.

As the GNC began to assume more responsibility for mental nursing, membership of the Society fell away. In 1947, there were 93 members, but 2 years later, the numbers had fallen to 56. In 1972, when the Society was wound up, it was felt that there was no longer a need to have a separate organization for mental nurses because of the more open policy adopted towards them by the GNC.

6.6 TRAINING OF MENTAL NURSES

Training was seen by the Society of Mental Nurses as the most important means of transforming mental nursing into a profession with high standards and high status. In 1941, two years after the establishment of the Ministry of Health, the first Chief Nursing Officer, Dame Katherine Watt, was appointed to head its nursing division. She had a staff of nursing officers one of whose jobs it was, although none had any experience of mental nursing, to oversee the process of absorbing the Board of Control into the Ministry. In January 1946, a working party was set up under the chairmanship of Sir Robert Wood to identify and confront the problems facing the nursing profession. The working party's brief was to investigate the proper role of the nurse and the training he/she needed for that role. The committee found that there was a wastage rate from all branches of nurse training of up to 54%; this was attributable to insensitive hospital discipline, long working hours, poor accommodation and recreational facilities, dissatisfaction with training, inadequate arrangements for the care of nurses' health, and the amount of domestic work students were expected to undertake.

The working party recommended a new scheme of training that would identify the training needs of students as distinct from the service needs of hospitals. It suggested that the organization of each School of Nursing should be the responsibility of a Director assisted by his or her own staff. Students should be supernumerary to the needs of the wards for 2 years, and in the first 18 months of training, general and mental nurse trainees should follow the same curriculum, branching off only for the last 6 months of training into their specialist fields. At the end of training, all successful candidates should be registered on a common Register.

It was hoped that by reducing the period of training to 2 years from three, by removing the restrictions placed on married staff, by developing a part-time nursing service and by making more use of male nurses, the problems of recruiting and retaining nurses might be overcome. Much of what the 1946 working party found and recommended was restated in subsequent enquiries.

6.7 TRAINING OF MENTAL NURSE TUTORS

Until the late 1940s, it was the norm for tutors to be general nurses with no experience of mental nursing. In some mental hospitals, doctors still did most of the teaching, and nurse tutors concentrated on such areas as first aid and the types of instruments used in surgery. The Society of Mental Nurses considered that tutors who intended to train mental nurse students should be expected to have practised in mental nursing and also to have followed a specialist teacher training programme which would enable them to meet the specific needs of these students.

There were few avenues open to nurses who wished to train as tutors. In the early 1920s, the League of Red Cross Societies set up an 'Advanced Course for Nurses' based at Bedford College in London, the only London college catering specifically for women. This course lasted for one academic year and nurses came from all over the world to follow it. It covered a wide range of topics including the history of nursing, principles of education and methods of teaching, ethics, social administration, social psychology, hospital management and school administration. The majority of nurses taking the Advanced Course were general nurses, but those who wanted to teach in mental hospitals attended lectures on psychopathology and mental hygiene at the Tavistock Clinic. Although it was the only course at this time which offered training specifically for nurse teaching, the GNC did not recognize it, claiming that the content of the course was weak because it did not include anatomy and physiology.

Another avenue through which nurses could become tutors was to take the Diploma in Nursing at London University. This course, inaugurated in 1923, focused on the history of nursing to 1919, the scientific basis and general principles of nursing, nursing ethics, and methods of teaching. Some lectures were given by psychologists who sought to apply psychology to mental nursing but, as with Bedford College's Advanced Course for Nurses, little time was devoted to those who wished to teach mental nurses.

Battersea College started a course for nurse tutors in 1932, and in the mid-1940s, this College, the RCN and Hull were recognized by the GNC as centres for tutor training. The GNC still did not regard the Advanced Course for Nurses or the Diploma as adequate preparation for teaching. The only requirement necessary for entry onto the official nurse tutor courses was registration on the general part of the Register. However, there were by now many doubly trained nurses who were presenting themselves for training and who returned as qualified tutors to teach nurses in mental hospitals. From the late 1940s, the number of general trained tutors teaching in mental hospitals began to decrease while the number of tutors with mental nursing experience steadily increased.

Nurse tutor courses were of one year's duration and the students were largely expected to finance themselves, with very little funding being available. One nurse who undertook the Tutor's Diploma at Battersea recalled his experiences as follows:

I was given a grant of £50 from the Ministry of Health when I did my tutor's course in 1948. The content of the course was the same for all nurses. The general nurses were in the majority, but the mental were by far the better qualified and the most experienced; some mental nurses had three nursing qualifications including experience during the war in the RAMC. Some of us could not afford to live for a year on that amount, so I washed-up and 'waited on table' at Lyons Corner House, Marble Arch, to enable me to exist and meet my expenses. The lecturers treated the mental nurses no differently from the other nurses.

Those who attended Battersea College were impressed by the friendliness of the place and the respect accorded to nurses. This respect was based on the fact that trainee nurse-tutors were mature students, experienced in their discipline, and generally highly motivated. Life-long friendships were forged at Battersea College and during the mid-1940s, the 'Old Bats' association was established which enabled tutors to meet after their courses were finished. Some of the 'Old Bats' were instrumental in founding the Society of Mental Nurses, while others went on to make considerable contributions to mental nursing, names such as Miss Olive Griffith, Betty Nicholas and Annie Altschul.

6.8 MENTAL NURSING DURING THE 1940s AS PERCEIVED BY MENTAL NURSES

The information which follows was gathered from 10 men and 10 women who entered mental nursing during the 1940s. All were retired at the time the interviews took place (1988), although a few were still working either part-time or voluntarily in a variety of mental health care community settings. The average age of the men had been 24 at the commencement of their training, and the age of the women 22; seven of the men had been single and three married. The men had all left school at age 14, but the women had generally had two further years of education. None of the women had been married at the time of entering mental nursing.

Some of the women had taken up nursing because of a long-standing interest in the work; the particular branch of nursing which they were to practise had not concerned them. Some stated that they had been attracted to mental nursing because it paid more than general nursing; for three interviewees, there had been a sense of inevitability about their choice of career as mental nursing was already 'in the family'. The women talked about how they had valued the order and routine of their work as nurses. They had enjoyed making wards homely for the patients and feeling themselves to be part of a larger family which was the hospital itself. They had taken great satisfaction from earning their own wages and thereby maintaining their independence. They also reminisced affectionately about the many friends they had made amongst their colleagues at the hospitals.

The men had had different reasons for becoming mental nurses. They had been partly motivated by the excellent sporting facilities provided at the mental hospitals. One respondent was adamant that these had been far superior to facilities then found at first division football clubs. All stated that the unemployment situation at the time had had some influence on their decision to take up nursing as the prospect of any job with a pension was enticing. Six of them had been deeply unsettled by the War, and the paramilitary atmosphere of mental hospitals felt comfortingly familiar. One had been told by a Medical Superintendent that his military background meant that he was already 90% trained. Another had had a religious conversion during the War and had made it his mission in life to care for disabled people after his discharge from military service. Two of the men had been brought up in the grounds of mental hospitals and felt that it had been natural for them to follow in the footsteps of their parents who were also mental nurses. One man was a farmer's son who had come into contact with mentally ill people as a boy when his father had employed 'peculiars' to help with the harvest.

Many of the men had been offered jobs at their first hospitals without an interview. Some had simply received a letter asking them to report for duty. Those who had been interviewed said they had generally been asked about what they could contribute to the hospital community. Although most of the men had considered mental hospitals as places run primarily for the convenience and enjoyment of the staff, some had valued their contact with the patients – talking to them, working with them, and seeing them get better. When working together on the land, staff and patients had often become particularly close:

There was tremendous companionship between staff and patients. Many of the patients knew far more about farming than the staff.

However, most of the men interviewed agreed that it had been the camaraderie amongst the staff which had kept them in nursing, and few had given any serious consideration to the needs of the patients.

The women interviewees made many adverse remarks about the harsh discipline prevalent in the hospitals during the 1940s, the poor food, and the low pay (£3. 10 s per fortnight) for the very hard work they had had to do. Having to apply for late passes had been a source of irritation to many. One nurse recalled being 3 minutes late, and having to endure the humiliation of a stern rebuke:

I arrived back at the hospital at three minutes past ten. I should have been back at ten. Next morning the Matron entered the ward where I worked and called my name at the top of her voice. I was told if I was ever late again I would be dismissed at once.

Not only was contact between male and female patients discouraged, relationships between male and female nurses were also frowned upon:

Meeting people of the opposite sex was difficult. . . . Because of the strict rules, sexual relations were rushed and so were marriages. Oftentimes marriages took place where the couple hardly knew each other. The result of this was that many marriages broke up, and there was a lot of marital infidelity.

The women recalled that there had been no incentive for them to improve themselves and that those nurses who had attended the twice weekly training lectures had been branded as 'work shy'. They had found nursing depressed patients a demoralizing experience as they had had no understanding of them and no training in how to relate to or care for them.

The male respondents gave detailed accounts of those aspects of mental nursing which they had found unrewarding:

I started mental nursing in 1947. I was given a cubicle at the end of a dormitory. When it was decided that I was useful, I was given a room. The last meal was at 4.00 p.m.; the lights were put out at 10 o'clock and we were up at 5.30 a.m. The Charge Nurses were in complete control of their wards and nobody ever challenged them. Many of them spoke in a bullying way to patients; they were arrogant and always spoke down to junior staff. They were men who were familiar with violence from the War. I was a coward – I should have done something about what I saw, but those to whom I would have had to complain were part of the same system. Patients who were beaten were seen by the Medical Superintendent who invariably accepted the account of the incident given by the Charge Nurse which was always untrue.

Even those male nurses who had not entered nursing primarily to care for the sick commented on the appalling treatment which the mentally ill had received during the 1940s. In some wards, patients had not been allowed to sing. Others had not been discharged even after making considerable progress; indeed, discharge policy appeared to have been entirely at the whim of the superintendent and there were many patients whom the staff considered completely sane who had not been discharged simply because they were good workers. The men mentioned other features of life in the asylums which had lowered the morale of both staff and patients:

Patients were subjected to hours and hours of endless boredom in the airing courts. It was soul-destroying for both patients and staff. Every time we went to or left the airing court, we counted the patients out and then counted them back. In the side-rooms, there were patients locked up for weeks on end; the staff had become so used to the screaming of these patients that they totally ignored it.

There were other duties which the respondents had not enjoyed, such as 'specialling' a suicidal patient. This meant that a nurse had to spend the entire night from 7.15 p.m. to 6.30 a.m. sitting with the patient, observing his every move to ensure that he did not come to any harm. The endless cleaning and scrubbing – on most wards, staff used 'bumpers' to polish and shine the ward floors three times each day – had been considered both futile and boring. One respondent remarked on the sense of unreality from which he had suffered when engaged in these chores:

It seemed as if we were marooned in time – nothing much ever happened, nothing much ever changed – and every task was repeated each day over and over again.

Keys had featured largely in the routine of the hospital and this emphasis on the custodial part of their duties had been distasteful to many of the male nurses. Staff wore belts with chains and keys attached. On being given his keys, one young man had been told:

Guard these with your life; if you lose them, your life won't be worth living.

The interviewees spoke of the embarrassment they had felt when asked by 'outsiders' what their job was. The women had claimed to be general nurses, or, that their work at the mental hospital was with patients with physical illnesses. Some of the men had suffered so much from an inferiority complex that they had preferred the security of the hospital community to meeting people from other walks of life. Relationships with girls from outside the hospital had frequently floundered:

> Whenever I met a girl and took her out, things went well until she asked what I did for a living.

Shortage of staff had been acute on the 'sick wards' where often there had been only three nurses to 75 patients. Under this pressure, the nurses had tended to vent their frustrations on the patients. Senior nurses had been remote figures who made unreasonable demands and caused resentment when they were not qualified; there had been instances of senior nurses having no nursing qualifications beyond a First Aid Certificate. Information about patients had not been available to the ward nurses and case notes had been kept in the 'central office' where only doctors had access to them.

Considering the hard labour involved in their work and the long hours on duty, the male nurses in particular thought they had been financially exploited. Low wages had prevented some from getting married. Career prospects had been poor. It took 25 years to become a Charge Nurse and promotion meant 'waiting for dead men's shoes'. There had been no opportunity to move from one hospital to another in search of better pay or conditions.

> When you trained in the 1940s, you trained for a particular hospital and that's where you were expected to stay. It was a sign of an awkward person if you left and applied to another hospital. In fact, there was an unwritten rule among superintendents that they did not poach staff from one another. If a member of staff wanted a job at another hospital, he was required to present a letter from his former superintendent to the effect that his services were no longer required.

In some rural hospitals during the War, it had proved so difficult to recruit nurses that Irish staff had been asked if they had relatives who would like to apply for posts. Superintendents and Matrons went to Ireland on staff-recruiting missions. The men and women they found took the places of nurses who had been called up for military service. After the War, when demobbed staff returned to their former hospitals, many had felt embittered. One nurse recalled:

> When I resumed my work as a nurse in the hospital where I had been prior to the outbreak of War, I was sorely disappointed. Many Irish nurses had been recruited during the War and were given Sisters' and Charge Nurses' posts. The most irritating thing about this was that they were not very good nurses. They mainly came from the West of Ireland, had little education and only a limited understanding of the mentally ill. Those of

us who returned found ourselves at the bottom of the pecking order and had to start all over again to build up years of experience before we got promoted.

6.9 MENTAL NURSING SKILLS IN THE 1940s

The nurses interviewed did not describe the work they had done in the mental hospitals during the 1940s as skilled. Many of them did not even know why they had been selected for nursing posts. Three types of people were described by the interviewees as having been representative of mental nurses.

6.9.1. Those with the Ability to Control

The power to control which some nurses had was described by the interviewees as a particular skill different from the aggressive posture adopted by the 'bullies':

The first Charge Nurse I worked with came from a family of attendants. He stood well over six feet tall. He walked in a deliberate and purposeful way and everyone knew he was in charge. When he entered the day-room, a sudden silence would descend on the place and all eyes turned towards him. He had a presence that I have never encountered in anyone else. If there was ever a fight among patients, he would stand by the door of the day-room and in a calm tone of voice mention the names of those involved and instantly the fight would cease. He would hold the offenders with his eye for five or ten minutes afterwards. I never saw him resort to violence; I would also say that the patients were not afraid of him. They respected him and they trusted him. They knew he was in charge.

Such nurses were described by the interviewees as having an instinctive understanding of mentally ill people. They abhorred violence and for the most part prevented it from occurring, but their wards were described more as being 'well run' than happy.

6.9.2. Those Who Controlled Through Fear

For some nurses who had had terrible experiences during the War, and who had received little or no support in coming to terms with those experiences, the War had continued on the wards where they had directed their anger onto the patients. Those whose control had been exercised through fear wanted their patients to be well-behaved and their wards to be always clean and tidy. Such nurses seem to have felt that the patients were in a conspiracy against them, and that staff must therefore assert their authority at all times.

Respondents who had worked on wards run by this type of nurse had quickly become accustomed to violence and had had to do things which they described as 'disturbing'. One nurse recalled that:

> There were certain wards where staff left very frequently, yet none of the senior staff ever attempted to establish why.

6.9.3. The Compassionate and Caring

The respondents talked admiringly of certain nurses who had been devoted to the patients, always calm, and blessed with a sense of humour. These nurses had been able to create an atmosphere in which people could be happy; they had taken an interest in new members of staff and had taken the time to explain the ward routine to them:

> He [the Charge Nurse] took me aside during the first week I was on his ward and explained to me what the work was all about. He told me that for some nurses, it was a mere job, but for him it was a vocation. 'It's something you must believe in. You must always do what is right because in the end right always prevails.'

Sensitive nurses of this type had appreciated that some of the patients were far more skilled than they in dealing with violence and epileptic fits, and in administering first aid to recalcitrant inmates. They had known the importance of being accepted by the patients as well as the staff:

> A Charge Nurse told me shortly after starting my training always to carry a 'baccy tin' (tobacco tin) in my pocket. You can get patients to do anything for a fag. Because I had been in the forces and was used to free cigarettes, I was a heavy smoker. The popular staff were the ones who gave fags to the patients. I had an added advantage in that I could cut hair, and whenever I went to do anything, about half a dozen patients jumped up to help me. Tobacco was a very powerful means of becoming accepted by patients.

The advice given by sympathetic Sisters or Charge Nurses had proved far more valuable to the interviewees when they had started nursing in the 1940s than the Sister-Tutors' lectures which had centred on the pathology of mental illness rather than on helping them to understand what they should have been doing in the clinical setting. The irrelevance of training was repeatedly commented upon by the interviewees. They had seen it merely as a means to passing their exams and so getting a pay increase.

6.10 THE 1950s: MENTAL HOSPITALS UNDER ATTACK

Jones (1991) presents the 1950s as an optimistic period for the mentally ill. New drugs came onto the scene in psychiatry; the open-door policy became established in mental hospitals and a Royal Commission was appointed to review the law relating to mental illness and mental deficiency. Although these events appeared progressive, and were certainly presented by doctors and government as being so, they occurred in a decade which saw not only innovation and critical enquiry, but also many contradictions and much opportunism.

During the 1950s, the tradition of caring for mentally disordered people within large institutions came under intense criticism both from inside and outside the system. The atmosphere within mental hospitals which had started to show signs of becoming more relaxed during the 1940s, changed considerably during the 1950s. There was a growing realization that the structure and organization of mental hospitals were essentially pathogenic; innovators in care demonstrated that new therapeutic ideas could be introduced into the existing system with beneficial effects. Thomas Main (1946) at the Cassel Hospital, David Martin at Claybury and David Clark at Fulborn were among the first to demonstrate that changing the organization of mental hospitals and adopting open-door policies could result in significant improvement in even the most institutionalized patients. Once the merits of an open-door policy had been clearly shown, more progressive superintendents were willing to follow suit and thousands of patients whose furthest boundaries had previously been the walls of the airing courts were liberated. At Warlingham Park, Dr Rees opened the doors of 21 of his 23 wards in the early 1950s; by 1956, 22 out of 37 wards were permanently open at Netherne Hospital and 60% of the patients were permitted unlimited access to the hospital grounds. Dr MacMillan opened the doors at Mapperly Hospital, Nottingham in 1954, Dr Stern did likewise at the Central Hospital, Warwick in 1957, and in the same year, Dr Mandelbrote opened the wards at Coney Hill Hospital in Gloucester (Rose, 1986).

It would, however, be wrong to consider that open-door policies and allowing patients some freedom completely dislodged more traditional ideas amongst doctors. The main duty of the mental hospitals was still, in the opinion of many medical practitioners, to provide humane custody of patients who were suffering from hereditary psychoses which would prevent their ever leaving the institutions (Clark, 1964). Rose observes that during the 1950s, tensions started to develop between traditional and more liberal-minded psychiatrists:

A fissuring was occurring in mental medicine. A certain hostility was growing between the long established sector of asylum superintendents, defenders of the need for separate and distinct institutions for the treatment of the mentally ill . . . and the physicians who sought the integration of the practice, training and facilities of psychiatry with those of the general hospital. (Rose, 1986)

Goodwin (1989) agrees with this analysis. He considers that those doctors who sought to transform the mental hospitals from within were essentially defending the principle of separate institutions for mental patients. These medical practitioners were not in favour of community care; what they supported was treatment in the community, but with the mental hospital remaining firmly at the centre of psychiatric services. Debate was generated by the uneasy recognition on the part of many practitioners of psychiatry that the profession was in the process of changing from a custodial to a treatment model of practice. Not only in Britain, but also in other countries such as Holland, the USA and Canada, psychiatrists were experimenting with a variety of new models of service provision.

6.11 INSTITUTIONAL CHANGE AND MENTAL NURSING SKILLS

For the most part, the history of psychiatry has been written by doctors; therefore the impression may have been created that all the many innovations which were introduced into the care of psychiatric patients during the 1950s were brought about by members of the medical profession. This distortion has probably been exacerbated by the fact that it was usual to associate mental hospitals with the names of their Medical Superintendents. Walk (1961) and Hunter (1956) have shown, however, that nurses played a significant part in effecting the changes which occurred during this decade; indeed some of them were nurse-led. Skilled nurses began to demonstrate that what they had to offer might achieve better results with patients than other forms of treatment.

During the 1950s, nurses, like doctors, began to recognize that the hospital atmosphere which forced inactivity upon patients and removed all responsibilities from them was hindering rather than helping their recovery (Cameron and Laing, 1955). Noisy and violent patients commandeered all the attention of the nursing staff, while withdrawn and solitary patients were habitually passed over and had very little personal contact with nurses or other patients. They sat around the walls, or lay on the floor, in the same place every day:

> Occasionally, one of them would attack another patient or a nurse, for no known reason, and then revert to her customary inactive state. If approached, several of them were liable to spit obscenities, or to attack. For this reason they were very seldom approached. (Cameron and Laing, 1955)

Although hospital life was not uniformly like this, and it is true that in some institutions, patients became friendly with the staff to the point where they helped out in the superintendent's house, played with his children, and did odd jobs for the staff, there were many hospitals where:

> A certain amount of personal danger and of involvement in degradation and brutality were accepted as inevitable if regrettable aspects of mental hospital work. (Clark, 1964)

Cameron and Laing (1955) reported that the transformation which took place at the Glasgow Royal Mental Hospital was started by nurses and patients spending time together. Nurses were allocated to the same patients each day and gradually the patients began to know them and relax in their company. Patients were encouraged to read, talk to each other and do things for themselves. After a short period it was noticed that:

> They paid more attention to their appearance, and some began to sew, draw, or make rugs. Most of them took over small jobs which they jealously insisted on doing for themselves. Thus, at tea-time, one patient made the tea, another laid out the cups, a third put the sugar on the table, another the milk, yet another spread the table-cloth, and so on. (Cameron and Laing, 1955)

The nurses responded warmly to the creation of an institutional climate where interpersonal relationships could be nurtured. Medical staff recognized that merely to provide materials with which patients could amuse themselves was insufficient without the input of the nursing staff. Nurses found their level of job satisfaction increasing (Cameron and Laing, 1955).

Similar results were being obtained at De La Pole Hospital, Willerby, in Yorkshire. There Dr Bickford, the superintendent, was generous in his appreciation of the improvement nurses were able to effect in the condition of even the most chronic patients. Bickford devised new, more patient-friendly routines for his nurses to implement:

> The patients were grouped in tens and slept, rose, washed and dressed, ate, played and worked in their groups, always having the same nurses with them. During the working day, they wore battle-dress. They had to keep this neat, their hair brushed, their shoes clean. They had to shave themselves like practically every other patient in the hospital. They had to wear a necktie except during hard work and games. At 4.00 p.m., they all changed into lounge suits. Each group had special duties each day. Every week, each group changed duties with another, so that their weekly routine was different for four successive weeks. The following is an example of what four groups could be doing on one day of the week:

Group 1:   a.m. Mess duties
              p.m. Bowling-green construction

Group 2: a.m. Bowling-green construction
           p.m. Country walk

Group 3: a.m. Educational discussion
                     Lacrosse
           p.m. Carrying ashes to bowling-green

Group 4: a.m. Bathing
           p.m. Educational discussion
                     Hockey

Lacrosse, tennis and hockey were considered suitable games for the patients because they were unfamiliar to most of them and, therefore, interesting and challenging. The educational discussions were arranged weekly in advance with nurses participating in selecting the topics for discussion. These included how to run a smallholding, chrysanthemum growing, dairy farming, the Liberal point of view, local government, the job of a cricket captain, care of a motor-bicycle, prospects for the Derby, and how to run a seaside boarding house. Every patient who came to these discussions was considered as having something worthwhile to say and even patients long regarded as 'chronic' were listened to with interest and respect. Bickford was able to report considerable success with his new regime, quoting the example of one patients who was initially so withdrawn that a psychiatrist had advised his mother to forget that she had ever had a son, but who was eventually able to go home regularly on leave. What was achieved at De La Pole Hospital indicated that much more could be done with chronic patients than had hitherto been considered possible; indeed many of them could return to the community.

During the autumn of 1955, Bickford organized groups of patients to go potato-picking on nearby farms. Patients and nurses enjoyed these outings in new surroundings; coach-rides and picnic meals made a pleasant change. For each day they worked, the patients gave 2 s 6 d to the hospital and the rest of the money paid by the farmer was divided between the pickers.

Many progressive hospitals in the mode of De La Pole Hospital owed their reputations and successes to a mixture of charismatic Medical Superintendents and enthusiastic nurses. Bickford's skills were complemented by the commitment of his Chief Male Nurse, Mr P. Archer, whom Bickford always singled out for special praise. Not all hospitals had the right mix of personnel to enable them to implement new and creative regimes, and, unfortunately, many of the progressive ones fell back into outdated and disabling practices when a particularly liberal Superintendent or dynamic Chief Nurse left.

6.12 THERAPEUTIC PROGRESS OR PHARMACEUTICAL HYPE

Baruch and Treacher (1978) argue that, having opted for a medical outlook on mental disease, psychiatry has inevitably tended to consider any drug that can be shown to alleviate symptoms such as anxiety or depression as efficacious. The alacrity with which psychiatrists have generally welcomed new drugs and treatments has been equalled only by their uncritical acceptance of the claims of drug companies and their lack of rigour in observing the side-effects of drugs. In reviewing insulin coma therapy, psychosurgery, electroconvulsive therapy and drug therapies, Baruch and Treacher (1978) contend that there was a general failure to conduct even the simplest trials to confirm their usefulness.

Eysenck (1952) was one of the first in Britain to point to the uncomfortable truth that the recovery rate amongst neurotic patients was unrelated to whether or not they had received psychotherapeutic treatments. He was closely followed by Bourne (1953), a junior psychiatrist, who, defying his own establishment, questioned the effectiveness of insulin coma therapy. Four years later, Ackner *et al.* (1957) confirmed his opinion that insulin did not have the therapeutic benefit it was claimed to have.

The customary tone of uncritical acceptance of new therapies continued, however, to be in evidence when the discovery of a major new drug was announced in 1952. Two French researchers reported the beneficial effects of Chlorpromazine (Largactil) in treating psychotic patients and in 1954, clinical tests tended to support their conclusion that it was useful in controlling psychotic excitement (Anton-Stephens, 1954; Charatan, 1954). For psychiatrists, it would appear that the prestige of having in their armamentarium a drug such as Chlorpromazine was sufficiently beguiling to allay any fears as to its possible side-effects. To be able to claim access to a drug which could 'cure' mental disease in the same way as doctors in other disciplines had their own range of curative drugs, was immensely attractive to those psychiatrists who felt that their scientific credibility would thereby be enhanced. Their enthusiasm was unabated by the Chief Medical Officer's 1954 Report which stated that it had not been possible to substantiate the curative effects originally claimed for the drug. His attitude was one of caution, claiming that it was far too early to assess the effectiveness of Largactil and its derivatives, as so little was known about the causes and nature of mental illness.

Aubrey Lewis, addressing the first International Conference on Neuropsychopharmacology in 1958, emphasized that non-interventionist approaches to care, such as ward activity programmes and occupational therapy could produce results comparable to those of Chlorpromazine. Clark (1964) later argued that the milieu in which drugs were prescribed was as important as the drugs themselves; drugs would have a more powerful effect if used within a therapeutic community setting. Only when coupled with sensitive nursing care would drugs realize their maximum potential in the treatment of psychotic patients. Smith, Kline and French, the manufacturers of Largactil, obviously agreed with this and considered it important to target nurses in their marketing programme. In association with the famous American nurse, Hildegard Peplau, the company produced a film aimed at nurses, made at Greystone Park Psychiatric Hospital in New Jersey. The nurses there enthusiastically endorsed the drug and the film was subsequently shown to student nurses in Britain. Smith, Kline and French claimed that by relieving patients of anti-social symptoms, they would become more open to the particular psychotherapeutic skills which nurses had to offer (Smoyak, 1991).

6.13 THREATENED EROSION OF NURSING SKILLS

Although nurses were central to pioneering work being carried out in various parts of the country during the 1950s, they were not as a group party to the wider debate about treatments which was taking place outside the mental hospitals, nor within their hospitals did they generally participate in case conferences, discuss patients' diagnoses or treatments, or assess the progress of patients. As a rule, they were unaware that what passed for treatment in their place of work might represent no more than the predilection of their particular medical superintendent, based on no firm evidence at all. Most nurses accepted that their role was to carry out uncritically whatever medical staff had ordained.

Hunter, however, was fearful that chemotherapy and physical treatments for psychiatric patients would diminish the mental nursing profession. He questioned whether nurses were becoming mere dispensers of medicines and assistants to doctors in the administration of treatments, and foresaw that their numbers might be so reduced that eventually they would cease to have any impact on care at all:

> Physical treatment replacing shortage of nurses starts a vicious circle of fewer nurses, more restraint disguised as physical treatment, less nursing, fewer nurses, more restraint and so on. (Hunter, 1956)

Nurses' jobs were also under threat from another source. During the 1950s, carers from two new disciplines began to assume direct responsibility for mental patients; these were social workers and occupational therapists whose numbers were increasing greatly. Should this trend continue, claimed Hunter (1956), the mental nurse would at worst be spending his/her time polishing floors, and at best, be merely a servant to the doctors. Hunter saw the skills of the mental nurse being valued far below those of the general nurse, and his/her status and conditions of work becoming ever poorer.

6.14 MENTAL NURSING: IN DECLINE?

In the early 1950s, articles began to appear which addressed the working conditions of the mental nurse. An Editorial in *The Lancet* in 1954 (p. 953) warned of an impending crisis. Nurses, it claimed, should be awarded 'danger money', not because of any threats posed by violent patients, but because of the appalling environment in which they had to carry out their duties.

A Royal College of Nursing conference in 1954, addressed mainly by doctors, discussed the 'staffing problems in mental nursing', and tried to analyse the reasons for low morale within the mental nursing profession. The conference heard that up to 80% of entrants to mental nursing left before completing their training (*Nursing Mirror*, 1954, pp. 1055–56 and 1193). Although a 15% increase in the nursing work-force in British mental hospitals had been announced in 1950, this increase comprised only untrained staff. Dame Russell-Smith, Under-Secretary to the Minister of Health, spoke of the reasons which might lie behind the high turnover of staff. She cited nurses leaving the profession for family reasons and because they found themselves to be unsuited to the work, but also, and very significantly, because of low pay, poor working conditions and inadequate teaching and training.

Job satisfaction was poor because of overcrowding in the mental hospitals, lack of co-operation between doctors and nurses, insensitive hierarchies which devalued nurses, nurses being used as domestics, inadequate remuneration and the demoralization which came from working with patients labelled 'incurable'. Training was largely irrelevant to the practice of mental nursing as it failed to address strategies for the case of mental patients. At least 15 months of the training were devoted to general nursing care and tutors often had little or no experience of psychiatric nursing. The conference concluded that mental nursing was in crisis and that certain recommendations should be implemented immediately:

1. Mental nurses and general nurses should be brought together under one nursing umbrella. By so doing, middle class females would be attracted into mental nursing, thus raising the standing of psychiatry.
2. The age of entry into mental nursing should be reduced to 17½, while the upper age limit should be raised to 60.
3. Teaching should be undertaken in small groups.
4. More co-operation between ward staff and tutors, and between doctors and nurses should be encouraged.
5. Psychology and sociology should be included in the nurse training curriculum and nursing staff should have the opportunity to see how patients could be cared for outside the hospital environment.

6.15 THE 1959 MENTAL HEALTH ACT

While the Royal College of Nursing conference was putting forward these strategies for ameliorating the crisis within mental nursing, the Ministries of Employment and Health had reached the rather different conclusions that the way forward was to employ more nursing assistants to ease the over-crowding in the mental hospitals and to look for alternative methods of caring for patients outside the institutions. Despite open-door policies and therapeutic community schemes, the population of mental hospitals had continued to soar so that by 1955 there were over 150 000 patients in mental hospitals, an expansion which, if allowed to continue, would have threatened the viability of the National Health Service. Because doctors and adminis-trators seemed unable to stem the rising tide of patients, the Government intervened with the 1959 Mental Health Act which was intended to reduce the number of in-patients immediately and, in the long term, to change the course of mental health care provision. The Act implicitly condemned overcrowding as an organizational malpractice productive in itself of a great deal of ill health. The assumptions underpinning institutional care were challenged again by introducing the concept of 'informal' patients who were to be treated in the same way as those with physical conditions, namely in out-patient clinics, by GPs and in the community. The impetus for the Act was doubtlessly economic, but it also took account of and embodied the dissatisfaction which had been mounting for years amongst those concerned with the plight of the mentally ill.

REFERENCES

Ackner, B., Harris, A. and Oldham, A. J. (1957) Insulin treatment of schizophrenia – a controlled study. *Lancet*, **2**, 607–11.

Anton-Stephens, D. (1954) Preliminary observations on the psychiatric uses of chlor-promazine (Largactil). *Journal of Mental Science*, **100**, 543–57.

Barnes, E. (ed.) (1968) *Psychosocial Nursing*, Tavistock, London.

Baruch, G. and Treacher, A. (1978) *Psychiatry Observed*, Routledge & Kegan Paul, London, p. 50.

Bickford, J. A. R. (1955) The forgotten patient. *The Lancet*, **1**, 917–19.

Bourne, H. (1953) The insulin myth. *The Lancet*, **2**, 964–8.

Cameron, J. L. and Laing, R. D. (1955) Effects of environmental change in the care of chronic schizophrenics. *The Lancet*, 1384–1386, 31 December.

Charatan, F. (1954) An evaluation of chlorpromazine (Largactil) in psychiatry. *Journal of Mental Science*, **100**, 882–893.

Churchill, W. (1951) *The Second World War*, Vol. 4, Cassell, London.

Clark, D. H. (1964) *Administrative Therapy*, Tavistock, London, p. 32.

Elles, G. (1968) *Psychosocial Nursing* (ed. E. Barnes), Tavistock, London.

Eysenck, J. (1952) The effects of psychotherapy: an evaluation. *Journal of Consulting Psychology*, **16**, 319–24.

Fisher, J. W. (1948) *Modern Methods of Mental Treatment – A Guide for Nurses* (Introduction), Staples Press, London.

Goodwin, S. (1989) Community care for the mentally ill in England and Wales: myths, assumptions and reality. *Journal of Social Policy,* **18**, 27–52.

Hunter, R. (1956) The rise and fall of mental nursing. *The Lancet,* **1**, 14 January.

Jones, K. (1991) The culture of the mental hospital, in *150 Years of British Psychiatry 1841–1991* (eds G. E. Berrios and H. Freeman), Gaskell, London, p. 25.

Main, T. (1946) The hospital as a therapeutic institution. *Bulletin of the Menniger Clinic,* **10**, 66–70.

Ramon, S. (1985) *Psychiatry in Britain: meaning and policy*, Croom Helm, London.

Rose, N. (1986) Psychiatry: the discipline of mental health, in *The Power of Psychiatry* (eds P. Miller and N. Rose), Polity Press, Cambridge, p. 59.

Smoyak, A. S. (1991) Psychosocial nursing in public versus private sectors. *Journal of Psychosocial Nursing,* **29**, 6–12.

Titmus, R. (1950) *Problems of Social Policy*, HMSO, London.

Walk, A. (1961) The history of mental nursing. *Journal of Mental Science,* **107**, 1–17.

Webster, C. (1985) Nursing and the early crisis of the National Health Service. *The History of Nursing Group at the RCN*, Bulletin 7, London.

7

Mental nursing in the 1960s and 1970s

7.1 INTRODUCTION

The seeds of community and out-patient treatment which had been sown in the 1950s were nurtured during the next decade when the Government's determination to reduce the number of beds in mental hospitals became quite clear. The ideology and practice of institutional care came under critical scrutiny, and the very existence of the mental hospitals was questioned. There were some who proposed that responsibility for psychiatric patients should be entirely removed from the National Health Service and given to Social Services. The implication seemed to be that patients were to be transferred from the control of doctors to the care of social workers and community psychologists (Ministry of Health, 1962). Indeed, large numbers of social workers were employed at this time to provide a service for ex-mental patients (Jones, 1988), and between 1964 and 1975 the number of psychologists employed in mental hospitals and in out- and in-patient units increased 10-fold (Busfield, 1986).

Neither social workers nor psychologists had any strong institutional allegiance, unlike psychiatric doctors and nurses, and they had no vested interest in preserving psychiatry within the institutions. Some considered that this made them better qualified to manage and deliver social care. They were to be part of a multidisciplinary approach to care for psychiatric patients, an approach which it was hoped would flourish when the less restrictive atmosphere of the community replaced the tightly controlled medical culture of the mental hospital. The quality of therapeutic interventions was expected to improve in the community and redress the bad practices associated with over-use of medication which suppressed symptoms, but ignored their causes and did nothing to enable patients to return to their everyday lives.

To transfer all patients from the hospitals to the community was not, however, immediately feasible given the very large numbers of patients currently occupying beds in mental hospitals and the fact that the organization of effective community care had scarcely begun to be addressed. It was the acutely ill patients who were ideally suited to the new environment of psychiatric care; they could receive short-term therapy in hospital and be speedily discharged back into the community; no one, however, had any real idea about how the long-term chronically psychiatrically sick were to be managed away from the institutions.

The influx of psychologists and social workers into mental health care and the growing influence of the community idea did not mean that the centre of the stage had been vacated by the medical profession, even if there were professional and lay groups who would have liked to see that happen. Doctors maintained their supremacy over the care of psychiatric patients (Baruch and Treacher, 1978). Nurses, however, were as little considered or consulted during the initial moves towards patient care in the community as they had ever been. Their centrality to the running of the hospitals was repeatedly overlooked and their experience disregarded. It was apparently forgotten that while the new community schemes were getting underway, the vast majority of nurses remained on the wards caring for the long-term sick who were not so easily displaced from the institutions. Nurses were not involved in any of the strategic planning relating to community care just as they were not involved in the community mental hygiene movement in the 1920s.

It seemed as if nurses were unable to respond to the threatened erosion of their role within psychiatry, an erosion which started in the early 1950s with the arrival of Largactil. The excitement this caused amongst medical practitioners was matched by apprehension on the part of some mental nurses who wondered whether psychotropic drugs might spell the end of nursing care for mental patients, or at least seriously reduce the need for nursing input. Hunter (1956) suggests that the introduction of drugs and the rapid escalation in their use accounts for both the deskilling and the demoralization of nurses which became apparent from the late 1950s into the 1960s; nurses felt that their therapeutic role had been reduced to giving out medications, and that both doctors and patients ascribed greater importance to drugs than to nursing care.

Meanwhile, as the new social scientists of the 1960s became interested in the organization and function of institutions, psychiatric hospitals found themselves under continued fire. Goffman's investigation into American psychiatric hospitals was both penetrating and critical and extended the work already begun in the 1950s by researchers such as Belknap (1956) and Dunham and Weinberg (1960). During his own long hospitalization with tuberculosis, Goffman gained personal experience of the effects of institutionalization and an interest in other people's experience of it. His study of psychiatric patients led him to conclude that mental illness was at least in part a creation of mental hospitals. He found that the social structure of mental hospitals resembled that of a 'total institution'. In such a situation, the staff's primary concern was to ensure that patients conformed; they achieved this by forcing inmates to enact their lives within a confined and observable space. Far from adhering to their original purpose of aiding mentally ill people towards recovery, the agenda in psychiatric hospitals had become solely the preservation of their own hierarchies.

123

Goffman's work *Asylums*, published in 1961, proved a landmark in the history of psychiatric care and for the anti-psychiatry movement of the period. The book was largely instrumental in bringing about a radical rethinking of care for the mentally ill in the USA and had considerable influence in Britain. *Asylums* found a visual counterpart in the film 'Snakepit' which was popular at the time and which depicted the most bizarre effects of mental illness.

In Britain, Barton (1959) had also recognized that many of the symptoms suffered by psychiatric patients were the effects of prolonged hospitalization. It was due to his influence that such therapeutic practices as 'habit training' and 'remotivation' became widespread in the 1960s. Barton developed the theme that the ideology behind the mental hospitals and the practices dependent on that ideology were more likely to inhibit than facilitate treatment. He was in no doubt that psychiatry was long overdue for a radical overhaul and noted that the many patients who were being discharged without having participated in social rehabilitation programmes were at grave risk of being readmitted, victims of their institutionalization. Barton's conclusions were addressed to all those involved in the care and treatment of the mentally ill, but nurses found themselves at the sharpest end of his book's criticism because of their close involvement in patients' daily lives.

7.2 GOVERNMENT PLANS AND NURSING MORALE

The first public acknowledgement by the Government that psychiatry was under scrutiny came from Enoch Powell as Minister of Health at the annual conference of the National Association of Mental Health in 1961. Mental hospitals, he stated, were part of a bygone age and these 'doomed institutions' must disappear. He predicted that of the 150 000 beds then available, only half that number would remain by 1975. He impressed upon his audience:

This is a colossal undertaking, not so much in the new physical provision which it involves, as in the sheer inertia of mind and matter which it requires to be overcome. There they stand, old type asylums, isolated, majestic, imperious, brooded over by the gigantic water-tower and chimney combined, rising unmistakably and daunting out of the countryside – the asylums which our forefathers built with such immense solidity. Do not for a moment underestimate their powers of resistance to our assault. (Powell, 1961)

What was required in order to remove them, he argued, was a completely new approach to the mentally ill and their welfare.

On 31 May 1961, Powell officiated at the opening of a Nurse Training School at Littlemore Hospital near Oxford. Again he emphasized the

Government's intention to cut the number of psychiatric beds, especially on long-stay wards. He stressed that this was not part of a campaign to undermine psychiatry; on the contrary it would strengthen it. More resources, he continued, would be spent on improving the training of mental nurses, and this would lead to an improved standard of care for patients. He saw nurses as having the opportunity to play a leading role in the 'exciting changes that lay ahead'. Those who chose mental nursing as a career could look forward to lives of variety, movement and challenge, far more rewarding and adventurous than the careers of their predecessors:

> Nowhere in the whole range of medicine is that scope larger than in the career of mental nursing which those who attend this school will have chosen. (Records of the Association of Chief Male Nurses)

Twenty-seven years later, when he reflected on the conditions in the Health Service at the time he gave his Littlemore speech, Powell (1988) commented that the mental hospitals had become so entrenched in their bureaucracies that it had been difficult to contemplate even the modest changes of which he had spoken. He had had access to no accurate figures on staffing levels and costs; lines of accountability had been non-existent or blurred. Nurses were spending most of their time on trivial domestic chores and were overtrained for such a role. He had known that without the driving forces of adequate finance and the good faith of staff, any plan, no matter how attractive, would fail from lack of a sense of urgency or direction.

The spirit of optimism Powell generated among nurses at Littlemore was short-lived. Despite his upbeat political rhetoric, mental nurses were not convinced that their lot was likely to improve. The Records of the Association of Chief Male Nurses (1953–74)[1] show that the atmosphere at their annual conference in 1962 was sombre, and dismay was expressed by a number of participants because of a more recent statement by Powell which apparently contradicted what he had said at Littlemore. Powell had remarked:

> It is not always necessary, nor always desirable, to have qualified staff supervising psychiatric patients. (Records of the Association of Chief Male Nurses)

The nurses attending the conference were suspicious of the Government's motives, and wondered whether its real aim was to reduce spending on psychiatry whilst appeasing nurses with the promise of improved status. They felt betrayed by the repeated attacks on psychiatry and nursing because they believed that changes had occurred in mental hospitals, that the welfare of

---

[1]These records are currently in the possession of Mr John Green who was a regular attender at these meetings. The records are to placed in the Royal College of Nursing library.

mental patients had improved, and that nurses had played a significant part in bringing these changes about:

> Paper by the ton and ink by the gallon has been used since the War in efforts to break down the fear and prejudice towards mental disorder held by the general public. Open days, nursing exhibitions, public meetings and sometimes a sympathetic press, all have played their part.

> While there has been a change outside hospital, a process of change has been evolving within. Rules like strict segregation of male and female patients have disappeared, unlocked wards are commonplace, and week-end leave is almost routine. In fact, it would be fair to say that there are fewer restrictions than in general hospitals. (Records of the Association of Chief Male Nurses)

However, the *Nursing Times* Editorial of 22 March 1963 did not support the claim that nurses were changing the face of psychiatry. It regretted that little was being done either to improve the standard of care for psychiatric patients, or the morale of nursing staff. The editorial suggested that the policy of employing unqualified staff to work on the wards might be the cause of the mental hospitals' problems:

> During the past ten years, there has been an increase of 3,629 untrained nursing assistants, but an increase only of 166 trained nurses.

Rubenstein and Lasswell's (1966) research into how nurses were perceived by patients confirmed the gulf between staff and patients which Goffman had identified 5 years earlier:

> The nurses were clearly regarded as part of the opposition . . . against whom the patient struggled to maintain his dignity, privacy and integrity. Nurses were always about at regular intervals during the night, awakening patients, nagging about getting dressed for breakfast, collecting laundry, serving meals, writing endless notes, handing out medications, enforcing rules and calling the doctor. (Rubenstein and Lasswell, 1966)

The study also found that most qualified nurses were happy with the rigid nature of the hospital hierarchy; they saw mental illness solely as a medical problem and were content to acknowledge the supremacy of doctors and their own subservient status.

Nonetheless, the tone of the 1964 conference of the Chief Male Nurses' Association was despondent. Delegates heard that 70% of student nurses left before completing their training. There were better job prospects elsewhere. Conditions of service within nursing, such as split shifts and being given duty rotas at very short notice, were anti-social and insensitive. In one hospital, a male nurse could have a day off to be the best man at a wedding, but not if he was the bridegroom! Training was irrelevant to the work of the mental nurse and took second place to staffing the wards. Psychiatry was being paralysed by conflict between nursing and medical staff and under threat from the Treasury which was adamant that further monies would not be forthcoming.

The pessimism of the conference found an echo the same year in Peter Townsend's article, 'Prisoners of Neglect', published in *The Observer* of 5 April. Townsend claimed that conditions within mental hospitals were unacceptable in a civilized country. He did not apportion blame either to hospital staff or to administration, but suggested that society at large had a duty to confront the problem. The article was the forerunner of many similar accounts which appeared in the press over the next two decades. Most nurses recognized the validity of Townsend's analysis of mental hospitals, but felt powerless to do anything about it:

What can nurses do about the appalling conditions that still persist in mental hospitals? . . . Nurses are asked to remedy the situation. How can they, when they have no power in the organisation and have no presence on any decision making committee? (Records of the Chief Male Nurses Association Conference 1964)

7.3 DEFINING MENTAL NURSING

For over a century, doctors and nurses had worked together within the institutions, and, for the most part, had done so without friction. Each group knew its role and place and the boundaries between the two, if not laid down in statutes, were well understood by all concerned. Once the institutional system of psychiatry began to come under attack, however, both groups and particularly nurses, wanted to define their role and its importance more clearly. When independent observers began to look at what was happening in the mental hospitals, and at whose door their shortcomings could be laid, nurses were urged to explain themselves and their professional activities. At this point, nurses started to analyse how what they did was different from what doctors did. This represented a major step in the relationship between the two professions and in the development of a separate nursing identity.

In the mid-1950s, mental nursing became the focus of a number of studies which examined different aspects of the nurse's work. In 1954, the Liverpool Regional Hospital Board looked at the nature and status of mental nursing (*The Work of Mental Nurses*), and 2 years later, a similar study was undertaken by the Manchester Hospital Board (*The Work of the Mental Nurse*). In 1955, Oppenheim and Ereman examined the role and training of mental nurses and their work was carried on by Maddox in 1957 and by John in 1961. All these studies reached the same conclusions: that mental nursing was a complex activity which was difficult to define, and that some aspects of the work of mental nurses had only the slenderest claim to be related to patient care.

The 1954 Liverpool study found that the hospital operated under conditions of chronic staff shortage which was worse on the female side than on the male side. The decline in nursing staff was most evident in the student nurse grade. In 1938, there had been 194 students, in 1953 there were 28. Students in training at the time of the study constituted only 10% of the nursing staff. Approximately two-thirds of students withdrew from training in the period 1948–53. Nearly all were recruited as nursing assistants and 'persuaded' to train. No minimum educational standard was required of them and no selection procedures or diagnostic testing were carried out. Students who showed a lack of basic linguistic and numerical skills during the first few weeks of training were demoted to nursing assistants again. Little or no formal instruction was given on the wards; by and large, nurses adhered to the view that skills could not be taught, but could only be acquired through practical experience. The study concluded that better dovetailing of academic work and ward teaching, and greater involvement of students in the clinical and therapeutic aspects of patient care would help to retain both students and younger staff. Better selection of students and a proper training programme for nursing assistants would, in the long term, help to alleviate the chronic shortage of staff. The Manchester study came to similar conclusions, although it felt that much of the work of the mental nurse could be carried out by untrained nursing assistants (MacGuire, 1969).

By the late 1950s, the emphasis had shifted from defining the role of mental nursing to examining the personalities and attitudes of those engaged in it. Gallagher *et al.* (1957) found that nursing assistants were likely to take on authoritarian roles and to distance themselves from patients, and in 1960 Menzies took up this idea when she found that task-orientated nursing fragmented care, so ensuring that nurses did not have to take responsibility for their actions, and were not accountable for individual patients. Staff who did not have the knowledge, the skills or the organizational support necessary to cope with very disturbed patients were thus protected from their own emotions and from professional accountability:

[Nurses] have constructed a social system which defends the practitioner from anxiety. Elaborate rituals have been devised in order to distance the nurse from the emotional life of the patient. Detachment from the job is achieved through routinisation of simple self-care tasks, and personal responsibility is taken out of the hands of those delivering care, thereby providing enough distance between the doer and the one who takes responsibility for all sorts of blame transference to take place. (Menzies, 1960)

7.4 MENTAL NURSE TRAINING IN THE 1960s

In the early 1960s, student general nurses from St Bartholemew's, King's College Hospital and Hammersmith Hospital started to be seconded to the Maudsley Hospital for periods of 8 weeks. The aim was to help them develop skills in forming relationships with patients, and it was considered that such skills might best be acquired with patients suffering from mental rather than physical illnesses. It was unquestioningly assumed that the ability to relate to psychiatric patients could be transferred to general patients and that experience in psychiatry would make students more effective as general nurses. More students from general hospitals were seconded to psychiatric institutions during the 1960s and 1970s until this became common practice. The 1968 Government Report 'Psychiatric Nursing Today and Tomorrow', questioned whether the reverse practice of seconding mental nurses to general hospitals was valuable. The Report found that far from increasing the flexibility of mental nurse students, this practice tended to diminish it.

The Report was sceptical about the environment of psychiatric nurse training. Were psychiatric nurses, merely by virtue of working in a mental hospital, or general nurses, merely by virtue of being seconded to them, therefore bound to develop interpersonal skills? One critic remarked acidly that there was a considerable distance between knowing what had to be done and being able to do it, and Martin (1968) felt that students needed guidance in forming therapeutic relationships rather than merely being put in the company of mental patients:

Nurses are well trained in the technical aspects of nursing and in the formal etiquette, but little or no help has been given in the past in the understanding and management of human relationships. And yet, this is probably the most essential qualification for the modern mental nurse. Without such training, nurses have constantly to fall back upon a rigid authoritarian system in order to maintain their security and status. They need the authority of the institution in order to clarify their dealings with their patients. (Martin, 1968)

Caine and Smail (1968) observed that nurses working in a therapeutic community setting put much less emphasis on physical treatments and the need for discipline than nurses working in traditional settings who believed that the smooth running of the institution took precedence over the individual needs of patients.

Student nurses did not have access to any literature which defined good nursing care and were not required to analyse their work. They therefore modelled themselves on the practices they saw employed on the wards. The theory they acquired was quite separate from their clinical work as the tutors who taught them anatomy, physiology, hygiene, psychology and the practice of nursing never visited the wards and did not see it as their job to do so.

If students were to receive the help they needed to learn how to form relationships with patients, trained members of staff would have to absorb new ideas and implement new patterns of care. The hospital culture itself and strong opposition from staff unwilling to abandon it precluded this from happening. Martin analysed the reasons for male nurses in particular resisting any challenge to the *status quo*:

> The male nurse tends to settle down in hospital, marry and build a home. Any apparent threat to his promotion prospects therefore strikes economically at the roots of his security and his home life. For this reason alone, he has a much stronger resistance to change if he feels it runs contrary to the approved policy of senior nursing staff on whom his promotion depends. (Martin, 1968)

The General Nursing Council realized that if training for mental nurses was to have any credibility in the 1960s, it would have to include some content on caring for mentally ill people in the community so that nurses could understand this new aspect of their role. The Council was able to appreciate that caring for patients outside the institutions would be very different from traditional patterns of care. In an attempt to meet the needs of nurses and patients in the community, the 1964 syllabus of training for mental nurses was introduced to include sociology, psychology and social psychology. For the first time, it was suggested that student nurses should spend some time outside their hospital on community placements. This represented a major break with traditional mental nurse training which had been geared solely towards training nurses within and for institutions.

7.5 THE EXPERIENCE OF NURSES DURING THE 1960s

A first-hand account of mental nursing during the 1960s was obtained from eight female nurses and 10 male nurses who started their training in British hospitals during that decade. These nurses had been aware that new ideas were coming into psychiatry and that the nurse training syllabus was being adjusted to accommodate them. An experimental syllabus had been introduced in 1957 although it was not fully adopted on a national scale until 1965. This syllabus recommended that mental nurse students should no longer sit for the preliminary examination which both they and general nurses had hitherto taken together, but should have their own specially designed examination paper.

Those interviewed had also been very aware of the 1959 Mental Health Act, although, in practice, its major impact appeared to them to have been confined to condemning staff nurses to hours of sifting through patients' records, crossing out the word 'Certified' and inserting 'Informal' in its place.

Only a few staff had taken up the spirit of the Act and responded to the patients' change of legal status by allowing 'informal' patients more freedom.

The nurses interviewed recalled the ever-present and generally glaring contradiction between what they were being taught as students and what they had seen happening in clinical practice. Staff, trained and untrained, showed very little willingness to meet the individual needs of patients; nursing care tended to be patronizing and disabling, so that patients became unable to perform for themselves even the most basic acts of day to day living. Rough handling of patients was common and concealed from senior personnel by general agreement amongst clinical staff.

The impact of research on psychiatry and psychiatric nursing during the 1950s and 1960s did not result in unanimity of thought and practice amongst psychiatric institutions. Hospitals varied in their theoretical stances and treatment modalities; even within the same hospital, different approaches to patient care could be found from one ward to another, or on the same ward depending on which nurses were on duty and which Consultant on call. Staff accepted that they treated each patient according to the individual preferences of his Consultant, and happily contradicted what they did with one patient by adopting a totally different approach towards another under the care of a different Consultant:

> Consultants differed very much in how they described mental illness and even more so in the treatment they prescribed. They believed ardently that their approach was right and to us nurses, whatever approach was adopted, they claimed to get results.

The interviewees, however, were keen to set against this depressing backdrop those instances where nurses had done pioneering work in the interests of the profession and of their patients. It would be a mistake, they felt, to presume that the inability to identify and implement good practice was endemic in mental hospitals in the late 1950s and 1960s. There were nurses and doctors who, dissatisfied with their own and their patients' treatment, attempted to change the system. These carers rebelled against Victorian attitudes which ignored the individuality of clients, and which found it therapeutic to segregate male and female patients even at church services, dances and concerts! They challenged the facelessness of mental hospital care and developed genuinely therapeutic relationships with patients. One interviewee recalled what he had observed as a young student in the early 1960s:

> In the hospital where I trained, all the patients were known to the staff. It did astound me how skilful staff were at assessing the mood of particular patients, and how they were able to cope with even the most truculent of patients. Of course, I saw bad practices but they were the exception and I preferred instead to concentrate on the more agreeable side of mental nursing. I saw individualised patient care at its best and that was twenty

years before it became fashionable to write about it. Many years later, I came to appreciate that I had trained at an exceptionally good hospital. (Johnson, 1991, personal communication)

In another hospital, a Charge Nurse and three staff nurses 'helped to get rid of insulin therapy' which was a twice weekly routine. Patients were selected indiscriminately and continued to be treated despite the lack of any evidence to suggest that their condition was improving either in the short or long term. It was a courageous move on the part of the nurses to suggest that such 'therapy' should be stopped. Conflict with medical staff had become heated as the doctors argued that it was the Consultant's responsibility to prescribe treatment and the nurses to provide unquestioning care. The nurses had referred them to the current controversy regarding the therapeutic efficacy of insulin. Eventually, insulin therapy stopped but relationships between nursing and medical staff remained strained.

One interviewee told how a staff nurse at his hospital who had recently returned from general training set about devising care plans for patients in 1962. Soon all the staff on his ward were participating in individual patient care based on care plans. This was considered very progressive and tutors from the School of Nursing brought students to observe the 'new method of nursing'. The nurses on the ward decided to request permission from the Consultant to file their 'nursing notes' in the same folder as the medical notes. The Consultant responded angrily and tore up the nurses' care plans in front of them, commenting that the patients were his responsibility and that he and he alone would keep any records that were needed. This incident caused an uproar; senior nurses supported the doctors; the tutors supported the ward staff, and medical and nursing staff were at each other's throats. Within a month, the staff nurse who had initiated the new scheme left the hospital.

All the nurses interviewed recalled incidents of theft, mostly perpetrated by senior nursing staff who had access to patients' property and food. Patients' money was frequently stolen as one respondent recalled:

The Assistant Chief Male Nurse would take the money round his wards on Friday afternoon, and the Charge Nurse on each ward would sign for the amount due to each patient. The Assistant Chief would only hand the money over to the Charge Nurse and never to anyone acting up. Later that evening, the Assistant Chief would return to the wards for his slice of the share out. Some money was used to buy cigarettes and sweets for the patients, but the rest was divided between the two Charge Nurses and the Assistant Chief.

Because of the ease of misappropriating money from elderly patients, it was considered very desirable to get a Charge Nurse's post on a geriatric ward. The sole ambition of some nurses was to be promoted to one of the 'back wards' and then to remain there until they retired. Some Charge Nurses were able to lead luxurious lives far beyond the reach of senior nurses – with new cars, holidays in the USA, and a box at Epsom racecourse – all on the illegal proceeds of their nursing posts. Although it had been common knowledge where their money came from, questions were never asked, and such criminal dishonesty simply became part of the folklore of the hospital.

Hoarding was also common amongst senior staff. The interviewees had seen cupboards full of butter, sugar, jam, cigarettes and sweets to which only the Charge Nurse or Sister had the key, and yet patients were frequently denied these commodities. Ward staff seemed to believe, like their 19th century predecessors, that stealing food was a perk of the job. The attitude still persisted that patients were not entitled to any luxuries and that their property belonged to the hospital and thus to the nurses working there. Hoarding was also a hangover from the war years when there had been great shortages, and even though these were now a thing of the past, staff still took delight in competing amongst themselves to see which wards could boast the largest hoards.

The younger nurses starting out on their training in the 1960s and the recently qualified came from a generation which had grown up with rapid social change and who were prepared to challenge the older nurses about their attitudes towards patients and staff. Inevitably, conflict resulted. There was an enormous resistance to change within the mental institutions as the student nurses had soon realized. They had found that their Schools of Nursing were either unwilling or unable to support them when they complained about staff stealing from patients, and that senior nurses were reluctant to upset the *status quo* by backing younger staff against more experienced staff even when cruelty to patients was at issue. One interviewee described the subtle threats to which new staff were subjected:

> It was my second week on the ward, and one morning the Charge Nurse and the Staff Nurse took a patient who was 'edgy' into a side room and beat him up. I was asked to come along and observe. It was a particularly nasty incident and one that I was not prepared for. When it was finished, the Charge Nurse turned to me and said, 'You never saw a thing, did you?' and I knew that if I ever mentioned what I had seen, they would simply have denied it.

Several interviewees talked about the arrogance of trained staff who, although they had little power within the institution as a whole, wielded a sometimes tyrannical sword when it came to running the wards and managing the lives of patients. Senior nurses had also tended to patronize para-medical staff such as occupational therapists, physiotherapists and psychologists who were just beginning to appear in the hospitals. Student nurses had found that new ideas about treatment and care were never put into practice. Instead, drugs and electro-convulsive therapy (ECT) continued to hold pride of place in psychiatry and nurses were, as they had always been, merely custodians of understimulated, bored patients:

> The two most common treatments were medication and ECT. . . . The 'good patients' helped on the wards and behaved themselves; the rest either idled their days away on the wards or went to occupational therapy. . . . Patients who did not get on well with the staff spent their time on the wards either smoking or watching television and that was the majority on most wards.

7.6 THE SALMON REPORT

The recommendations of the Salmon Report on Nursing Management (DHSS, 1966) were eagerly welcomed by psychiatric nurses. The Report created a better career structure for them, doubling the numbers of those in management largely by creating a new post of Nursing Officer. Nursing Officers had a role to play in clinical supervision, management and personnel work, and although many who were appointed to the post had had relatively little experience of and no formal education in management, it was expected that they would change the face of nursing. However, this increase in the number of nurse-managers was never evaluated and it is impossible to say what contribution, if any, was made by Nursing Officers to improving nursing practice. The Salmon Report did increase mobility amongst the nursing work-force and psychiatric staff became less likely to remain at the same hospital for their entire career. Management positions were open to outside competition and promotion in the psychiatric hospitals was no longer a question simply of 'waiting for dead men's shoes'.

7.7 THE ERA OF PUBLIC ENQUIRIES

The 1960s saw the plight of the mentally ill become a public issue and the need for action was moved up the political agenda. People from outside psychiatry began to ask why conditions within the mental hospitals had not improved:

> Psychiatry is a public property. It is like no other area of medicine – thought about, agonised over, discussed and criticised by people who have no direct contact with it as a medical discipline either as practitioners or sufferers. (Blakemore, 1981)

Some staff began to rebel and, despairing of changing the system from within, called upon influential outsiders to help. There was a feeling amongst psychiatric nurses that the many Reports on the mental hospitals had become mere 'stalling tactics' by governments which wanted to appear compassionate while spending as little money as possible on an issue that was unlikely to be a vote winner. Nurses and social workers in large numbers began to write letters to various prominent figures (Robb, 1967), resulting in a letter being published in *The Times* on 10 November 1963, signed by 10 of the recipients. The letter read:

> We, the undersigned, have been shocked by the treatment of geriatric patients in certain mental hospitals, one of the evils being the practice of stripping them of their personal possessions. We have now sufficient evidence to suggest that this is widespread. . . . We shall be grateful if those who have encountered malpractices in this sphere will supply us with detailed information, which would of course be treated as confidential.

The contents of the letters received by the 10 signatories became the basis of a book entitled *Sans Everything, A Case to Answer* (Robb, 1967). The book described the undignified suffering of elderly people in hospitals and showed that with a little effort, their situation could be improved. There were many to claim that the book was exaggerated, but it was highly influential and prompted closer scrutiny of the treatment of other vulnerable groups in care such as children, the mentally handicapped and the mentally ill.

Once hospital staff had realized that recourse to outside agencies could be more effective in redressing the wrongs of the institutions than invoking the authority of senior nurses, the tradition of secrecy within the mental hospitals was broken. A nursing assistant wrote to the Sunday paper, the *News of the World*, which specialized in sensational criminal cases, condemning the treatment of patients at Ely Hospital in Cardiff. The information was forwarded to the Minister of Health and the unattributed letter was published on 20 August 1967. An all-party committee was set up and in 1969, the Ely Hospital Enquiry was published, the first of 18 subsequent public enquiries into the running of Britain's hospitals. The Ely Report substantiated many of the claims made by Robb, finding evidence of cruelty to patients and pilfering of their food, and indifference to such malpractices on the part of senior nursing management, medical staff and the Physician Superintendent. Similar findings, some worse, were made in the course of enquiries at other hospitals (Martin, 1984). Behind the compassionate rhetoric of psychiatry and the efforts of the Salmon Report to empower nurses to regulate their practice through the Nursing Officers, the enquiries revealed an inability either to recognize or to act on the gross deficiencies of the mental hospitals.

The criticisms directed at nurses during these enquiries were noted by the General Nursing Council (GNC) and impelled the Council to reconsider its approach to nurse training. Training still remained theoretical, based on a knowledge of diseases and types of treatments. Practical examinations were conducted in 'practical rooms' within the Schools of Nursing; students laid up trays and trollies and gave verbal accounts of how procedures would be carried out, but there was no assessment of their handling of patients. The result was that qualified nurses found themselves unprepared for the clinical environment and often unable, or not allowed, to practise what they had learned.

The GNC decided that the emphasis on training must be shifted so that learning in the clinical context became the priority. By 1972, assessments of students were ward-based with clinical staff acting as examiners. The Council's attention moved away from the Schools of Nursing. The effect of this, combined with citations made during the public enquiries, meant that by 1977, 57 out of just over 100 Schools of Nursing were under threat of closure (Johnson, 1991, personal communication). This revolution in training gave priority to enabling students to relate to patients in a therapeutic manner; their progress was measured by continuous assessment. So ended the era of theoretical teaching and examinations.

These changes within psychiatric nursing were part of a cataclysm by which the whole of the nursing profession was affected, so that within two decades, Schools of Nursing had disappeared to be replaced by Colleges of Nursing and Departments in Polytechnics and Universities. Nursing students became full-time students pursuing a career through higher education. They were no longer employees attached to a particular hospital, but students in the process of becoming highly qualified professionals who, it was hoped, would transform a modest service into one of exceptionally high standards.

7.8 MENTAL NURSING IN THE 1970s

In 1975, the year by which Enoch Powell had predicted that mental hospital beds would have been greatly reduced, the Government published a report entitled 'Better Services for the Mentally Ill' (DHSS, 1975) which evaluated the current state of the psychiatric services and outlined a plan of campaign for the future. Successes were detailed including less overcrowding in hospitals, more patients being treated and the rising number of patients being cared for in the community. Failures too were identified; staffing levels were still too low, and community facilities inadequate. The Report recognized that public tolerance would be stretched if ex-patients were not properly supported and supervised in the community. It also stated that no mental hospitals had been closed and that, for the foreseeable future, the hospital would remain at the centre of the mental health services. However, the Report noted that pressure on hospitals to discharge patients quickly, coupled with little support for them in the community, meant that 'revolving door patients' were becoming a feature of inadequate psychiatric care.

In the introduction to the Report, Barbara Castle, Secretary of State for Social Services, stated that mental illness constituted the most important challenge to those concerned in contemporary health and that community care was the best approach to the problems of mental illness. Although the

Report made no attempt to define exactly what community care meant, there was an assumption that an ideal service would be based on the 'primary care team' consisting of the GP, the health visitor, the district nurse and the social worker. The specialist therapeutic team would remain hospital based, covering in-patients, out-patients and day patients (Jones, 1988). No reference was made to how or when additional funding would be made available to local authorities to enable them to set up community care services, nor was there any mention of training staff in skills which could make community care effective. It seemed that the community care directive was essentially politically and economically inspired because no pilot studies into its management or effectiveness were ever conducted. The Report could not refer hospitals and local authorities to any literature which might show them how to proceed, although it reminded them that if community services were not properly co-ordinated, they would prove disastrous.

As the build-up of psychiatric services in the community got underway during the 1970s, it became obvious that nurses needed training and education to support them in making the transition from the hospital to the community. The first course for Community Psychiatric Nurses (CPNs) in the UK was well established at Chiswick College by the early 1970s, and similar courses became available throughout the country shortly afterwards. By the end of the decade, CPNs were starting to gain recognition as independent practitioners; they were working within general practices of health clinics in much the same way as health visitors, or accepting referrals from other agencies (Simmons and Brooker, 1990). Nurses were acquiring specialist skills and dealing with specialist groups, a different experience for them entirely from working in mental hospitals.

Nurses were also starting to analyse their skills by undertaking their own studies into psychiatric nursing. The conclusions of such studies were very much that the rhetoric of community care and its good intentions hid many drawbacks which were not being addressed. A number found that nurses were not skilled in establishing and maintaining interpersonal relationships and had no theoretical basis upon which to stand when caring for mental patients. Altschul (1972), Towell (1975), Cormack (1976), Clinton (1981) and Pollock (1982) lay much of the blame for this at the door of nurse education which they found still to be institutionalized, and likely to produce nurses who sought the security of institutionalized practices, avoiding opportunities for innnovation. The work of these researchers stimulated wide-ranging discussion and closer examination of nursing practices, and the amount of research activity undertaken by nurses grew steadily (Pollock, 1989).

REFERENCES

Altschul, A. (1972) *Patient-Nurse Interaction: a study of interactive patterns in acute psychiatric wards*, Churchill Livingstone, Edinburgh.

Barton, W. R. (1959) *Institutional Neurosis*, John Wright, Bristol.

Baruch, G. and Treacher, A. (1978) *Psychiatry Observed*, Routledge & Kegan Paul, London.

Belknap, I. (1956) *Human Problems of a State Mental Hospital*, McGraw-Hill, New York.

Blakemore, C. (1981) The future of psychiatry in science and psychiatry. *Psychological Medicine*, **11**, 27–38.

Busfield, J. (1986) *Managing Madness*, Unwin Hyman, London.

Caine, T. M. and Smail, D. J. (1968) Attitudes of psychiatric nurses to their role in treatment. *British Journal of Medical Psychology*, **41**, 193–7.

Clinton, M. (1981) Training psychiatric nurses: a sociological study of the problem of integrating theory and practice. Unpublished PhD Thesis, University of East Anglia.

Cormack, D. (1976) *Psychiatric Nursing Observed*, Royal College of Nursing, London.

Department of Health and Social Security (1966) The Report of the Committee on Senior Nurse Staffing Structure, HMSO, London.

Department of Health and Social Security (The Salmon Report), (1975) Better Services for the Mentally Ill, Cmnd. 6233, HMSO, London.

Dunham, H. W. and Weinberg, S. K. (1960) *The Culture of the State Mental Hospital*, Wayne State University Press, Detroit.

Gallagher, E. B., Levinson, D. J. and Ehrlich, I. (1957) Some socio-psychological characteristics of patients and their relevance for psychiatric treatment, in *The Patient and the Mental Hospital*, Free Press, Glencoe.

Goffman, E. (1961) *Asylums*, Doubleday & Co, Anchor Books, New York.

Hunter, R. (1956) The rise and fall of mental nursing. *The Lancet*, **1**, 14 January.

John, A. (1961) *A Study of the Psychiatric Nurse*, E. & S. Livingstone, Edinburgh.

Jones, K. (1988) *Experience in Mental Health. Community Care and Social Policy*, Sage Publications, London.

MacGuire, J. (1969) *Threshold to Nursing*, Occasional Papers on Social Administration, no. 30, G. Bell & Sons Ltd, London.

Maddox, H. (1957) The work of mental nurses. *Nursing Mirror*, **105**, 189–90.

Martin, D. V. (1968) *Adventure in Psychiatry*, Bruno Cassirer, Oxford.

Martin, J. P. (1984) *Hospitals in Trouble*, Basil Blackwell, London.

Menzies, I. (1960) The functioning of the social system as a defence against anxiety. *Human Relations*, **13**, 95–121. Reprinted as Tavistock Pamphlet 3 (1970).

Ministry of Health (1962) *A Hospital Plan for England and Wales*, Cmnd 1604, HMSO, London.

Oppenheim, A. M. and Ereman, B. (1955) *The Function and Training of Mental Nurses*, Chapman & Hall, London.

Pollock, L. C. (1982) *Learning to Relate*, Royal College of Nursing, London.

Pollock, L. C. (1989) *Community Psychiatric Nursing: myth and reality*, Royal College of Nursing, London.

Powell, J. E. (1961) Speech by the Minister of Health, the Rt Hon. Enoch Powell. Report of the Annual Conference of the National Association for Mental Health, London.

Powell, J. E. (1988) My years as Health Minister. *The Spectator*, pp. 8–10, 20 February.

'*Psychiatric Nursing Today and Tomorrow*' (1968) Report of the Joint Sub-Committee of the Standing Mental Health and the Standing Nursing Advisory Committees, HMSO, London.

Robb, B. (ed.) (1967) *Sans Everything: a case to answer*, Nelson, London.

Rubenstein, R. and Lasswell, H. D. (1966) *The Sharing of Power in a Psychiatric Hospital*, Yale University Press, New Haven.

Simmons, S. and Brooker, C. (1990) *Community Psychiatric Nursing: a social perspective*, Butterworth-Heinemann, London.

Towell, D. (1975) *Understanding Psychiatric Nursing*, Royal College of Nursing, London.

8

Mental nursing in the 1980s

8.1 THE NHS IN THE 1980s: ECONOMICS AND MANAGEMENT

Between 1948 and the mid-1970s, the NHS underwent enormous expansion. Successive governments were keenly aware of the cost of the ever-increasing demands of the Health Service, but the NHS had become for the British a birthright and any party proposing cuts risked a serious loss of votes at election time. The expansion was therefore allowed to continue until the economic crisis of the 1970s forced the Government's hand (Clay, 1987). In the words of the 1979 Royal Commission on the NHS:

> The NHS could not shelter from the country's chill economic climate in the mid 1970s.

Where the 1960s in Britain had been a period of economic prosperity with relatively little unemployment, by the 1980s, unemployment had reached nearly three million, the economic base of the country was less robust than it had been two decades before, and there was increasing reluctance on the part of Government to fund the public sector.

The Government calculated that the economy of the country could not support an ever more costly Health Service. The principle of free health care for all at the point of delivery was much cherished by the British public and envied throughout the world, but new sources of funding had to be considered. The crisis in the NHS was witnessed by long hospital waiting lists and ward closures. Patients were being denied sometimes life-saving treatment because of lack of resources. The media covered poignant stories of children in need of heart surgery and unable to obtain it at the Birmingham Children's Hospital. In this instance, television was influential in prompting the release of extra funds to provide nurses to staff the intensive care unit at the Hospital. The underlying crisis, however, remained.

The Labour Government of the 1970s had not envisaged major structural alteration to the Health Service, but Conservative Governments of the 1980s found the NHS inefficient and bureaucratic. Their aim was to introduce 'market forces' which would make the Health Service more accountable to the public and give better value for money. A philosophical and practical transformation of the NHS was initiated. Health managers and carers were encouraged to embrace industrial principles of practice with the emphasis on cost-effectiveness, and to abandon the model of service which had persisted for over 40 years. In 1982, Area Health Authorities were abolished. Competitive tendering arrived in 1983, particularly in the areas of domestic and catering services. Ideologies such as health promotion and self-help featured in circulars from central government and gradually began to be absorbed into the thinking and working practices of health professionals.

Hospitalization of patients came to be seen as a last resort. One way of reducing the cost of the Health Service was to close the long-stay hospitals or decrease the number of patients in them:

> The elderly, the mentally ill and the mentally handicapped were finally publicly noticed and the standards of care they received questioned. Was it really appropriate and cost-effective to keep people in the institutional environment of hospitals? The answer was clearly no, and the seeds of the policy of wholesale care in the community were sown – the full implications of which we are realising only now. (Clay, 1979)

Community care was intended by its proponents to imply a people-centred approach to health care rather than a professional-dominated one. Home life was to be preferred to institutional care, local services to distant ones, and the ideals to be pursued were those of normalization and integration. However, the House of Commons Social Services Committee (1984) heard that community care had become a term that was 'virtually meaningless'. For most Health Districts, it simply meant cutting their costs by getting people out of hospital. The 1986 Audit Commission for Local Authorities in England and Wales pointed out that despite the reduction in hospital beds, Social Services had received no extra resources to fund care in the community. The burden of care was falling on families and volunteers rather than on the statutory services. Many believed these findings confirmed that the driving force behind community care for those with mental health problems in Britain and the USA was not the pursuit of therapeutic efficacy, but what was politically and economically to the advantage of government (Smoyak, 1991).

Political critics continued to argue that the Health Service had become too bureaucratic and that consensus decision-making was too slow. The Griffiths Report of 1983 recommended the introduction of General Managers who would be empowered to set objectives and take decisions. It also considered that doctors should become more involved in management but, by failing to mention nurses, was by implication critical of their managerial abilities. Nurses' confidence was seriously eroded. Few nurses felt inclined to apply to be General Managers so that by the late 1980s, there were only three in post. A survey conducted by the Royal College of Nursing in 1985 found that one-third of Health Districts did not have a senior nurse, and suspecting that the profession was being belittled, mounted a vigorous campaign in the media against general management. General Managers were portrayed as 'not knowing their humerus from their coccyx', while in more muted tones, it was suggested that nurses did not know 'their debit from their credit'. The College considered that the new basic nurse training programmes with their emphasis on management skills meant that nurses would very soon be quite able to take their proper place in the ranks of managers.

8.2 TRAINING IN THE 1980s

The severity of the cut-backs in the NHS was felt by nurses in terms of staff shortages and lack of resources. The 1983 Mental Health Act granted mental nurses 'holding powers' to detain patients for up to 6 hours. This apparent regard by Government for the authority and status of mental nurses was also a cost-cutting exercise in that the Act devolved power to a professional group within the mental health service who were less highly paid and therefore more cost-effective than doctors.

In 1982, student wastage during training reached 35% (Judge Commission on Nursing Education, 1985). The Judge Report, spear-headed by an educationalist, found that there was a great need to improve staff morale at all levels and that the way to do this was to reform nurse education. The Report considered that the knowledge base of nursing should be considerably broadened so that students were 'educated' rather than 'trained'. Criticism was levelled at the close links between Schools of Nursing and hospitals which led to student nurses being seen as employees rather than as students. A broader knowledge base acquired within non-hospital-based schools was, the Judge Report argued, the prerequisite if nurses were to learn to cope with the multi-faceted problems of contemporary care both at a conceptual level and in the practical setting.

The Judge Report was in the same tradition as previous Reports which had, over the years, attempted to tackle the problems of recruiting and retaining nurses through training. It did not analyse what strategies might be needed to support nurses educated in the new way once they entered practice; it did not look at the training of senior management, or the problems of inter-professional rivalry, role confusion and duplication of effort. Many critics of the Report argued that there would be no improvement in nursing care until the attitude amongst nurses that theorists were members of an elite, and practitioners people dependent on routines which required little or no thought, had been overcome.

Nearly a century after the introduction of the first training scheme for mental nurses in 1891, a 'new' training syllabus arrived in 1982 which aimed to revolutionize the nature of psychiatric nursing in the UK. The 1891 scheme had appeared in the wake of institutional care; the 1982 Syllabus for England

and Wales appeared in the wake of a new philosophy which saw psychiatric hospitals as being self-evidently undesirable, an assumption often accompanied by an uncritical advocacy of 'community care' (Weller, 1989). Despite its claim to be 'new', many of the ideas contained in the syllabus were not, although an attempt was made to distance psychiatric nursing from mere role-modelling or rule following, and to encourage nurses to see nursing as an evolving profession (Bergman, 1983; Jolley, 1987). The process of deinstitutionalization being well under way, the syllabus aimed to help nurses develop skills appropriate to community settings and to their role as health promoters.

The General Nursing Council (GNC) was galvanized into developing the 1982 Syllabus by the publication of the Jay Report in 1979 (DHSS, 1979). This report had looked critically at the work of mental handicap nurses and had suggested that poor standards of care for mentally handicapped clients were partly attributable to the training which their nurses received. Those who cared for the handicapped required educational, psychosocial and community skills, and the Report questioned whether nurses were needed at all in the field of mental handicap. Many concluded that the Report intended criticism of the GNC for retaining hegemony over a group of people who were incorrectly described as nurses.

Immediately following publication of the Report, the Mental Nurses Committee at the GNC met to discuss fundamental changes to the mental nurses' syllabus. The urgency was indicative of an intention to pre-empt any of Jay's conclusions being applied to mental nursing. A group of experts was convened to write the syllabus which emphasized the acquisition of interpersonal skills in order to indicate that in future, nurses would work by themselves away from the security of the institution. The design of the syllabus signalled the end of institutional training and was seen as an assertion of professional independence by psychiatric nurses. Whereas the Royal College of Psychiatrists had been consulted when previous syllabi had been drawn up, on this occasion it was not.

Many of the assumptions on which the new syllabus was based were quite untested, namely that psychiatric nursing is a skilled profession, that nursing competencies can be learned, and that the skills cited in the syllabus would indeed enable patients to get well. The syllabus did not consider that whereas nursing had been central to the practice of psychiatry in an institutional setting, it was far from clear what place it would occupy, if any, in a community setting.

In the 1920s, changes in nurses' thinking about themselves had been embodied in new terms, with 'patient', 'nurse' and 'hospital' being preferred to 'lunatic', 'attendant' and 'asylum'. In the 1980s, nurses began to favour the title of 'therapist' and to discuss the 'therapeutic relationship' the 'therapeutic environment' and the 'therapeutic process' to which the syllabus saw them as being central and not, as they had always been led to believe, peripheral. The widespread adoption of social and psychological models of care and treatment during the 1970s and 1980s enabled the syllabus to claim that the input of nurses was of equal value to that of any other members of the therapeutic team.

The syllabus started from the premise that psychiatric nursing was essentially different from general nursing and that the psychiatric nurse was a different kind of practitioner from the general nurse. This position had been radically undermined before the end of the decade by Project 2000 which emphasized the similarities between general and psychiatric nursing and abolished direct entry into either branch. Instead, all nurse students were to undertake a Common Foundation Programme.

8.3 PROJECT 2000

Project 2000 aims to transform nurse education in the UK by the year 2000. It represents the most radical overhaul of training in the history of nursing, and was necessary, according to the United Kingdom Central Council (UKCC, 1986), in order:

- to win for nursing students the status and educational opportunities of other professional groups undertaking a vocational education;
- to terminate the practice of immersing students in hospital culture and ward routines;
- to establish links with Institutions of Higher Education so that nursing education might receive academic validation;
- to improve morale in the profession so that recruitment of the 30 000 new nurses required each year in the UK might be assured (bearing in mind the reduced numbers of young people coming onto the job market) and their services retained;
- to place greater emphasis on health promotion and disease prevention than hitherto.

Project 2000 envisages that the number of qualified nurses will fall markedly, but that the number of Health Care Workers will increase. These workers will undertake some aspects of the practical care of patients under the supervision of qualified nurses. Entry requirements to Project 2000 type courses are five GCSEs or the equivalent at Grade C or above. Mature students can sit the UKCC DC Test in order to gain entry. The term 'psychiatric nurse' is replaced by 'mental health nurse'.

Project 2000 recognizes the nursing process as a suitable framework for the practice of both general and psychiatric nursing. Within this framework, interpersonal and communication skills and the therapeutic use of self are seen as vital. This emphasis brings psychiatric nursing in the UK abreast of its practice in the USA where the importance of developing relationships was recognized as long ago as 1948:

During their training, each student met with one patient twice a week for a period of 16 weeks. These sessions were referred to as 'talking with the patients', so as to gain an in-depth understanding of psychopathology. They were, in reality, preparation for counselling, which in the 1960s was finally called one-to-one or individual psychotherapy. (Peplau, 1989)

At face value the recommendations contained in Project 2000 appear progressive and aimed at enabling nursing to realize the professional status it has so long sought. By facilitating improved status for nursing as a whole, mental health nurses hope their standing will rise along with that of their colleagues in other branches of nursing. The thinking contained in Project 2000 is in line with that of many Reports which have previously attempted to tackle the problems of nursing in general and of psychiatric nursing in particular. However, the Common Foundation Programme, although masquerading as a new phenomenon, is, in effect, a return to the old Preliminary Examination which had been taken nearly a century before by general and mental nurses at the end of their first year of training.

If the number of general nurses is to decline during the 1990s, so too will the number of mental health nurses, and it may be that, eventually, instead of having different types of nurse, all will converge in the figure of the generic nurse as is the situation in the USA and in most European countries. Project 2000 may hasten the demise of the mental health nurse as the individual contribution of such a health specialist becomes subsumed into the profile of the generally trained nurse. The driving force behind Project 2000 came from general nurses and it is clear that they have most to gain from it. In a political climate where a quick return on investment is essential, general nurses are seen as far preferable to mental health nurses whose work requires time and the effects of which are not easily assessed.

This brief analysis of the state of nursing in the 1980s is by no means comprehensive. The economic, political and professional angles are each multifaceted in their impact on the overall situation. In the final analysis, the position of nurses in the 1980s may best be encapsulated in the feelings and opinions of the nurses themselves working within a rapidly changing, often confusing and contradictory work situation. The study which follows took as its sample a cohort of student nurses in training from 1984 to 1987. These students were at the sharp end of the new thinking in psychiatric nursing; they were the guinea-pigs on which the new 1982 Syllabus tested itself. As newcomers to nursing, they were able to analyse what was happening in the Schools of Nursing and in the institutions objectively, bringing a fresh perspective to the nature and practice of psychiatric nursing in the 1980s.

Table 8.1 Sample demographic data

Category	Female	Male
Sample size	28	9
Mean age	24	25
Age range	18–38	19–33
Single	19	5
Married	8	2
Divorced	1	2

8.4 THE SAMPLE

A sample of 37 learner nurses who started their training in September 1984 in five different Schools of Nursing in the west of England was selected (Table 8.1). All the students were first level entrants. Three of the Schools were in urban and two in rural areas. Although it is not possible to generalize from such a small sample, the data derived provide a valuable insight into the thinking of learner nurses at a time when training believed itself to be changing radically.

All but two of the students lived near the hospital at which they were training. At the rural Schools, all the learners were local people, suggesting perhaps that in the 1980s, as in the 19th century, hospitals were still being seen as a source of employment opportunity.

Compared with national data for entrants into psychiatric nursing in England, the preponderance of female over male applicants is representative. National figures collected since the setting up of the UKCC in 1983 also reveal a gradual fall in the numbers applying to do psychiatric nursing (Table 8.2).

None of the Schools in the sample had a formal policy regarding the academic subjects they regarded as desirable for psychiatric nursing, although two would not accept Art, Religious Knowledge, Music or Domestic Science qualifications. Interviewers claimed that they considered educational achievements as but one factor in the assessment of an applicant's overall suitability and felt it important to take into account personality, references and 'life experiences'. Three women from the sample had no formal academic qualifications and were accepted via the ENB Entrance Test, an alternative mode

Table 8.2 Numbers applying to psychiatric nursing, 1984–90

Year	Male	Female	Total
1984/85	639	1426	2065
1985/86	626	1272	1898
1986/87	648	1182	1830
1987/88	770	1026	1796
1988/89	867	1107	1974
1989/90	803	1059	1862

Source: ENB Post-Registration Records

of entry into psychiatric nursing for mature students. This test examines mathematical, spatial, and verbal reasoning, but is not considered to have validity in predicting 'good psychiatric nurses' or attrition rates.

Between them, the learners held qualifications in 28 different subjects, mainly at 'O' level. The most common subjects offered were, in rank order, English Literature, English Language, History, Mathematics, Biology and Sociology. Seven of the sample were graduates and held degrees in Art (2), Psychology (1), Education (1), Librarianship (1), Philosophy (1), and Physical Education (1).

All 37 men and women in the sample had had work experience prior to commencing psychiatric nurse training. Some had had evening or weekend jobs while still at school. Those who had been in full-time employment had been nursing assistants, general labourers or clerical assistants, or in domestic or service work. Some had taken a reduction in pay on entering nursing, but the majority had not. Even those who were changing their career direction remained, for the most part, within the same income parameters. In a study of general nurses, Mercer (1979) concluded that those who had had jobs prior to taking up nursing were often not making as significant a career change as might at first appear. Nursing had many characteristics in common with their previous work, e.g. pay and conditions of service, companionship, level of variety of tasks and opportunity for career advancement.

8.5 REASONS FOR ENTERING PSYCHIATRIC NURSING

The majority of the sample justified their decision to enter psychiatric nursing on the grounds that they wanted to help mentally ill people and felt they had something to offer. Those who had previously held a succession of short-term jobs dismissed the suggestion that this could be interpreted as an inability to settle, justifying themselves rather as being able to adapt to a variety of situations.

Mercer (1979) argued that it is difficult to obtain valid information from subjects who are asked why they want to become nurses. When plied with such questions, people say what they consider to be acceptable; reasons such as 'I want to care for people', or 'I want to do something worthwhile' are given. The respondents may not be aware of their own motivation for entering nursing, or cannot articulate it. The reasons applicants have for applying to train may not be the same reasons for which they remain in nursing. During training, learners may rethink their reasons for choosing to become nurses.

When asked to analyse what influences had led to their decision to apply for psychiatric nurse training, 15 of the women in the sample said that they had been influenced by a female relative involved in nursing or ancillary work, while 22 stated that none of their family was involved in any work that could be classified as 'caring'. Amongst this group, reading about mental illness and seeing television programmes had caught the interest of some, while others knew of people suffering from a psychiatric condition. One woman attributed her desire to become a nurse to her 'over sensitiveness' and to her 'social conscience':

When I worked in a pub, I saw a cross-section of people. Those I really felt sorry for were the ones who came in just after opening time, asked for a half of shandy, sat by themselves and were still there at closing time. I have known one old gentleman spend the whole evening staring at the floor, totally oblivious to what was going on around him. On several occasions, he left the pub without even touching his drink.

These individuals intrigued me. I felt really sorry for them, but as I never had the time, I never found out anything about them. On many evenings, before closing time, the pub would be full of conversation, singing and laughing, and every now and then, two or three solitary souls would appear in my line of vision. Where did they come from? And where did they go at night time? What did they do all day? I bet in all the world there was not one person who knew the answers to these questions. I still can't forget those souls: they are desperately in need.

On the whole, the sample claimed that they wanted to become nurses in order to help patients and to feel that they were doing something useful. Only one stated that in order to be helpful, she felt she should first learn about psychiatric conditions. The men and women interviewed had, in general, entered nursing with preconceived expectations of what the work entailed and of what aspects would appeal to them. Many had brought into nursing, or very soon acquired, a number of negative attitudes about the work. Within a few weeks of starting training, students were vocal in discussing aspects of psychiatric nursing which they disliked such as caring for elderly people, giving drugs to confused patients, 'smelly jobs', working in Victorian asylums, low morale and looking after people who would never get better.

Why do students undertake training and continue with it if they have such attitudes towards nursing? Some may have made a decision to tolerate the less pleasing aspects of nursing until reaching a senior position where their work would be more agreeable, or in which they could exercise influence to change what they disliked. It may have been the case that some students had changed their jobs so regularly that they were simply giving psychiatric nursing a 'try'. Some of the learners may have found it difficult to get employment elsewhere and having been accepted for training, were going ahead in the hopes that nursing would prove more satisfactory than anticipated. Doubtless, some students had totally unrealistic expectations of what the work entailed, but despite disenchantment, considered it easier to go on than to withdraw.

8.6 NURSES' REACTIONS AT THE END OF TRAINING

Of the 37 learners who started training in 1984, two men and four women left before the end of the course. Three of the women left because they were dissatisfied with the work and felt their talents could be better used elsewhere; the fourth had become pregnant but did not envisage returning to nursing. One of the married men dropped out because he was unable to support his family on a student nurse's pay. The second male student abandoned training because:

It was not at all what I had thought nursing was about, nor was it what I had been led to believe. I was keen to help people, but there was too much emphasis on the importance of meetings and rules about what ought to happen, when in reality little got done.

8.6.1 Psychiatric Nurse Training: a Positive Experience

When invited to reflect on their training, only a few students had found it a useful and inspiring experience. These few felt they had grown as people, had developed a better appreciation of their work and looked forward to the future with optimism:

When I started training, I was shy and retiring, lacked confidence and would shrivel up at the thought of having to say something in public. Over the past three years, I have learned to work on my own, to speak for myself, and to argue and discuss points. I am not as gullible and accepting as I once was; I am now more discerning and critical. I do not think these changes would have happened in any other line of work.

8.6.2 Psychiatric Nurse Training: a Disturbing Experience

Eight of the sample stated that training had been a disappointment to them and working with the mentally ill 'a disturbing experience'. All intended to leave nursing:

Training has changed me. I have completed the course, but I have paid a price for it. The long hours of work, night-duty, unsocial hours, preparing for exams and taking home with me unfinished business has had its toll on my marriage. I now live apart from my wife and children. I am cynical, unhappy and regret that I ever started training. As soon as I get the results of my exam, I will leave nursing for good in order to preserve whatever sanity I have left.

Another respondent commented in a similar vein:

Training, I feel, has exploited my good will. I have spent long periods close to sad and depressed patients, using the skills I have been taught in School, but no one has given me any support. It appears to be assumed that learners can cope with all of life's crises, and should be able to look after themselves. Well, I can't.

Learners were disappointed by the unrealistic attitudes of tutors and managers who seemed to consider that new approaches to care were easy to implement. Some felt that senior nurses deliberately avoided finding out what was happening on the wards in order to protect themselves and avoid having to confront unsatisfactory situations. Tutors were under the mistaken impression that what they were teaching in the classroom could be put into practice in the clinical arena.

8.6.3 Psychiatric Nurse Training: a Confusing Experience

Over half of the respondents stated that their training had left them unsure about their role and status as psychiatric nurses, and without a knowledge base which would enable them to address the contemporary debate within nursing. They had become aware of the wider issues in health care and nursing, such as Project 2000, the Griffiths Report and community care; they knew the theory behind individual autonomy and health education; but they had not been enabled to see how these ideas related to psychiatric nursing or to their own careers. They had noted that the term 'patient' was falling into disuse while 'client' and 'resident' were being preferred. Some students wondered whether concepts of 'therapists', 'carers' and 'mental health workers' signified that the future of psychiatric nursing was uncertain.

The nurses accused all the disciplines involved in psychiatry of paying no more than lip-service to the idea of involving patients in decision-making about their own care. They had found many patients did not understand why they had been admitted to hospital, what treatment they were having or when they were going to be discharged. Even when patients were present at case conferences:

They were treated in the most abominable way. They were talked about as if they were not there and what they said was largely ignored.

The training programme was radically flawed according to the students in that they had discussed concepts of care and aspects of the psychiatric nurse's role which they had never seen put into practice. One nurse commented that the reality she had witnessed in the clinical arena had suggested to her that:

People do not behave towards each other, least of all towards the mentally ill, in the spirit of altruism that underpins most of the therapies.

150

The students criticized tutors' too ready acceptance of theories and models of care originating in other countries, but untested here. Project 2000 was attacked for its illogical philosophy of according learners supernumerary status so that they could spend most of their first year as observers on the wards:

> But if what is done now is wrong, how can nurses under the new scheme be expected to do things better by observing what is happening? Indeed, if learner nurses are removed from the work-force, inevitably standards will fall because in my experience, most practical nursing is done by learners.

8.7 CONCLUSIONS

Students who felt positively about their psychiatric nurse training were few in comparison to those who felt unhappy about it. The fact that 50% of the sample did not intend to remain long-term in psychiatric nursing and that eight planned to leave immediately after their exams, speaks for itself. This disturbingly high wastage of new recruits before they had even started to practise in a trained capacity was related to the conviction amongst many of the respondents that psychiatric nursing had no clearly defined aims or direction. In their opinion, radical alternatives to care were impossible because senior nurses had little power to implement change without the permission of doctors or of general managers. The hospital hierarchy appeared to the learners to be completely out of touch with clinical practice and unable to tolerate independent thought or practice. The spontaneity that ought to lie at the heart of interpersonal relationships was stifled by a routine which subjected everything, including patients and their welfare, to itself. Nurses were being strangled by senior nurses, by medical staff, by more assertive disciplines and by institutional routines.

Nurse tutors were heavily criticized both for their work in the classroom and for their absence from the wards. They were accused of being blind to the gulf between what they were teaching students and what was possible in practice. Students had found them unwilling or unable to support them when they encountered problems during clinical placements.

The respondents felt that morale amongst psychiatric nurses was very poor. Any improvement in patient care was being hampered by nurses' long anti-social hours of work and poor pay, and by the many members of staff, both trained and untrained, who appeared to be carrying out their nursing duties in a way very different from what either hospital policies or the Schools of Nursing advocated. Like their predecessors earlier in the century, learners had tried to adopt experienced ward staff as role models in order to find out what they themselves should be doing. Modelling was difficult, however, when most staff had little knowledge of or sympathy with the new syllabus and were entirely sceptical about new ideas and students' enthusiasm.

These were the views of a cohort of 1980s students who were generally far better educated than entrants in previous decades. They were critical, self-assertive, articulate and threatening, although the issues they raised were not new. They were issues which had been considered on many occasions in official reports and hospital enquiries through the 1960s and 1970s. After 3 years in training, these students had found that nursing practice and teaching were stuck in antiquated moulds. Their account of the state of psychiatric nursing was based on limited experience which disabled them from appreciating changes that were occurring in the long term. However, their very newness to nursing facilitated a clarity of approach to its problems which provided a valuable, if in some ways restricted, analysis of what was happening in the Schools of Nursing and in the clinical areas.

REFERENCES

Bergman, R. (1983) Understanding the patient in all his human needs. *Journal of Advanced Nursing,* **8**, 185–90.

Clay, T. (1979) Nurses – power and politics. *Nursing,* Heinemann, London, p. 13.

Clay, T. (1987) *Nurses – Power and Politics,* Heinemann, London, p. 14.

Department of Health and and Social Security (1979) *Report of the Committee of Enquiry into Mental Handicap Nursing* (Jay Report), HMSO, London.

Jolley, M. (1987) The weight of tradition: a historical examination of early educational and curriculum development, in *The Curriculum in Nursing* (eds. P. Allan and M. Jolley) Croom Helm, London.

Judge Commission on Nursing Education (1985) *The Education of Nurses: a new dispensation,* Royal College of Nursing, London.

Mercer, G. M. (1979) *The Employment of Nurses – Nursing Labour Turnover in the NHS,* Croom Helm, London.

Peplau, H. E. (1989) Future directions in psychiatric nursing from the perspective of history. *Journal of Psychosocial Nursing,* **27**, 18–28.

Smoyak, A.S. (1991) Psychosocial nursing in public versus private sectors. *Journal of Psychosocial Nursing,* **29**, 6–12.

United Kingdom Central Council for Nursing, Midwifery and Health Visitors (1986) *Project 2000: a new preparation for practice,* United Kingdom Central Council, London.

Weller, M. P. I. (1989) Mental illness – who cares? *Nature,* **339**, 249–52.

9

Past, present and future

9.1 INTRODUCTION

The Enlightenment created a climate in which philanthropists with a concern for the poor, the disabled and the disadvantaged could take up the cudgels on their behalf. Humanitarians such as Tuke and Pinel undertook pioneeering work on behalf of the insane and strove to change social attitudes so that the dignity and human rights of the mentally disordered could be acknowledged. Their efforts influenced physicians, politicians and legislators in their own countries and even farther afield with the result that institutions devoted to the care of the insane were established in many countries. By the beginning of the 19th century, the public sector had begun to assume responsibility for a group of people with special needs who had previously been the responsibility of the family, if of anyone. By the mid-19th century, a system of institutions had been set up and it was within these institutions that the medical discipline of psychiatry took root and developed.

Psychiatric nursing arose pragmatically once the asylums had been created. What was required in these institutions was not a highly-trained work-force, but rather one well versed in the Victorian values of hard work and self-control and used to labouring for little pay and in poor conditions. Asylums tended to recruit local labour from the farms in the rural areas where they were often built; they also drew upon people who had been in service to gentry and upon the ranks of the semi-skilled. These men and women expected to work hard and not to complain; they certainly did not expect to have any say in how they were paid or to be offered attractive career prospects. Male attendants were chosen for their physique and robust health so that they would be able to control aggressive inmates and protect female nurses and physicians. Unattractive as asylum work may have seemed, it provided employment for those who did not want to leave their homes to become part of the swelling urban industrial populace.

The organization of the asylums was similar on both sides of the Atlantic. Peplau describes the first asylums in the USA in words which could equally apply to institutions in Britain:

> The earliest model was hierarchical and more or less paternalistic. Many mental hospitals were, in effect, closed systems. They were self-contained villages which, like old manor houses in Europe, were self-sustaining communities, presumably regulated in terms of the 'good of the whole'. Patients were the workers, attendants and nurses the patient-custodial managers, while physicians prescribed the treatments and in many instances, the rules of conduct. The hospital staff for the most part lived within the compound and intermarriages (across levels of power and authority within the hospital) were common. (Peplau, 1989)

The daily routine of the attendants was not dissimilar from the life of servants in great country houses. What the attendants did in the asylums during these early years could not be classified as 'nursing'. Their role was more like a prison warder's than akin to that of nurses who worked in general hospitals. Many asylum superintendents chose, therefore, to employ demobilized soldiers as attendants, men to whom the giving and taking of orders and institutional life were already familiar. Routine and hard work were considered therapeutic in themselves, and discipline was the chief means by which it was hoped disturbed patients could be reformed into upright citizens. The attendants both orchestrated and participated in this highly organized existence. They were expected always to be busy as 'busy-ness' was considered synonymous with industry and efficiency. The work ethos of the new industrial factories with their long hours and lack of freedom for individual creativity and initiative suited the asylums equally well. It was not for factory workers or attendants to question what they were doing or to evaluate outcomes.

Indeed, the state of psychiatry in the late 19th century was so nebulous (for all the well publicized claims of the medical profession) that it would have been an uncomfortable task to satisfy any enquiring work-force as to the rationale behind asylum life and the treatments enforced on patients. From the point of view of asylum doctors, the hierarchy of the institutions with themselves at the top was best maintained if attendants' knowledge constituted no more than the lay person's perceptions of mental illness.

Consolidated within the institutions, the medical profession devoted its energies to the search for a 'scientific' understanding of insanity. Nevertheless, as the 19th century advanced, psychiatry achieved no greater success in the treatment of insane patients than what it achieved through patients' natural ability to cure themselves. In the meantime, the attendants were acquiring non-medical skills which grew out of a developing tradition of institutional care composed of the wisdom which was passed on from one generation of attendants to the next. Because attendants and patients lived in close proximity – sleeping in the same dormitories in some asylums – friendships developed which were based on an understanding that was substantively different from that which the medical staff claimed to have. The attendants often shared a common background with patients. There was a

154

cultural empathy between them, whilst doctors kept the bulwarks of 'science' and 'objectivity' solidly between themselves and their patients.

Because of the rapid turnover of staff in asylums, the attendants had to rely on patients to explain the ward routines to them. 'Good' patients who helped the staff and lent a hand with recalcitrant inmates were highly valued. Nobody wished to see them discharged, whereas apathetic and aggressive patients were eagerly moved on. The asylum system thereby found itself caught on the horns of a dilemma; its aim was to cure and discharge patients as quickly as possible, but at the same time, it had to remain self-sufficient through patient labour. Those patients most ready for discharge were the ones whose labour was most productive.

If 'healthy' patients were not to be discharged and young male staff to be kept under control, the asylums had to channel their frustrations in ways which would safeguard the regime. For many years, the asylum system effectively protected itself by providing first-rate facilities for sport, music and amateur dramatics. Inter-asylum football and cricket matches and athletics meetings united patients and staff in support of 'their team', thus generating loyalty to the institution. Asylum bands enabled staff and patients to express themselves creatively in a way that the monotonous routines of daily life within the institutions could not accommodate.

Sport, drama and music controlled staff and patients as effectively as the asylum rules and the 'Handbook' with which all attendants were issued. They facilitated staff and patients in identifying with their particular hospital and created a sense of solidarity. So smoothly did this system of checks and balances work within the asylum system that it eventually required little effort on the part of Medical Superintendents to enforce it. Superintendents were consequently freed to pursue other interests and some were absent from their asylums for long periods at a time.

9.2 THE IMPACT OF MENTAL NURSE TRAINING

When attendants started to be trained in 1891, psychiatry could boast no clear definitions of mental disorder or scientifically tested treatments, and there was certainly no generally accepted area of expertise called psychiatric nursing. The first training courses were therefore based on medical knowledge of first aid, and offered a pragmatic approach to handling difficult and aggressive patients. Such training was not designed to stimulate critical thought, but the fact of having undertaken a course of instruction inevitably led attendants to believe that they were skilled. The medical profession capitalized on training to improve its own public image by claiming that the increasingly detailed practice of psychiatry now demanded skilled assistants.

In effect, training attempted to provide in-service 'education' for the largely uneducated men and women who presented themselves as asylum attendants at the end of the 19th and beginning of the 20th centuries. It embodied the ethos of the institutions in that the didactic approach adopted by the medical teachers remained the message rather than the medium; nurses were expected to adopt a similar style in their dealings with patients. The nurses who undertook training considered it as a means of achieving higher status and better pay; they did not consider it relevant to the way in which they cared for patients. Nurses went on learning their work by observing and then imitating other colleagues and training, instead of bringing enlightenment often brought disenchantment because it raised expectations which the asylum system could not meet.

Psychiatric nursing in Britain remained largely separate from general nursing until the introduction of Project 2000 in the 1980s, a century after the Medico-Psychological Association's training scheme for attendants began. This was in contrast to what happened in the USA where, from the beginning, training for attendants was included as part of the overall effort to improve nursing staff in all fields of practice. American training schemes considered that the skills of psychiatric and general nurses, though different, were complimentary. Divisions between psychiatric and general nurses in the early days of nurse training in the USA quickly disappeared to be replaced by the concept of the 'generic nurse'. Most American general nursing schools offered classes and clinical experience in aspects of psychiatric nursing. Divisions persisted in British nursing, however, for over a century with Project 2000 representing the first serious attempt to bring the various branches of nursing closer together. It may be that the professionalization of nursing in Britain has been impeded by the lack of mutual support and co-operation which have long been characteristic of nurse practitioners in different fields.

9.3 FROM THE INSTITUTION TO THE COMMUNITY

In the 1920s, the mental hospitals became grossly overcrowded as the myriad victims of the First World War were admitted for treatment. Progressive ideas strove for expression in a daily reality of nursing work which was repetitive and unimaginative. The men and women who applied for nursing posts were those desperate for any kind of work at a time of high unemployment. Few were really interested in the patients. The emphasis within the asylums was still on conformity. Caring for patients well did not bring promotion; carrying out one's duties with alacrity and military precision was far more likely to attract the attention of superiors. Job satisfaction was minimal. Although some nurses developed therapeutic relationships with patients, lack of knowledge and motivation, coupled with poor conditions of service and low status resulted in a high turnover of staff.

In the 1940s, psychiatric nursing in Britain, still struggling with overcrowding and understaffing, remained largely a mixture of modified 'mother role' activities: discipline of patients and custodial companionship (Peplau, 1989). The 1950s saw psychiatric nurses becoming more involved in medical treatments, particularly the administration of drugs. The effect of this was to entrench them even more firmly in the institutions where drug therapy was now at the forefront of care. In the USA, on the other hand, some psychiatric nurses were already moving out of the institutions and becoming established in private practice as nurse psychotherapists. Unlike their British counterparts, American nurses were far quicker to seize opportunities which would allow them to develop skills leading to autonomy.

Throughout the 1960s and 1970s, the hitherto closed system of psychiatric care began to open up at an unprecedented rate on both sides of the Atlantic. The old order was unceremoniously denounced and dismantled as hospital farms were sold off; hospital bands, football and cricket teams ceased to play. In the 1980s hospital houses were put on the market and later Nurse Training Schools disappeared. Allegiance to a particular hospital was no longer fashionable and more and more nurses lived their social and domestic lives independently of their place of work. Such was the rate of change that many older staff experienced occupational disorientation and felt forced to take early retirement. The late 1980s and early 1990s have witnessed the phenomenon of psychiatric hospitals emptied of patients and sold to property developers. A few have preservation orders on them so it can be hoped that some of these often magnificent buildings with their fascinating insights into past attitudes and practices will survive.

9.4 TWENTIETH CENTURY THEORY AND PRACTICE IN PSYCHIATRY

An examination of the system of psychiatry in Britain suggests that the different professional groups working within it hold different beliefs about what they do and set out to achieve different goals. These professionals generally conceive of themselves as providers of a therapeutic and self-evidently benign service based upon a growing body of professional expertise and objectively validated, morally neutral, scientific knowledge. For them, ineffectiveness within psychiatry is compounded by inadequate funding, understaffing, competing philosophies of treatment, interdisciplinary rivalry and poor training. Psychiatry's more radical critics argue that real as these problems are, they do not constitute the whole problem and that it is the social role of psychiatry and the contradictions contained within it which undermine the genuine attempts of psychiatric professionals to help their patients (Handy, 1991).

The major contradiction within psychiatry is that it is simultaneously part of the regulatory superstructure of our society and a system of care which aims to alleviate personal distress, some of it iatrogenic. To provide therapy for troubled individuals while at the same time controlling them for society's good is a conflict that most nurses have difficulty in resolving. What are the rights and responsibilities of the mental health patient and to what extent should staff feel empowered to make decisions for them?

> On the one hand, cultural norms concerning mental illness highlight the concept of unintelligibility and lack of responsibility, while on the other hand, norms concerning appropriate sick role behaviour give patients a clear duty to comply with medical treatment. This ambiguity can allow psychiatric patients to behave in a socially unacceptable manner and then deny responsibility for their actions, while simultaneously giving staff a mandate to deny the validity of the patient's perspective whenever it conflicts with their own goals. (Handy, 1991)

With these issues still requiring clarification, psychiatry is taking upon itself an ever-broadening spectrum of responsibilities; no longer content with the task of treating mental illness, it also aims now to identify subtle behavioural problems below the level of frank deviancy which it claims require the expertise of mental health professionals. The general public, while disillusioned with the mental health care system, has been persuaded that psychiatric professionals should be called in to deal with all minor mental aberrations. As long ago as the 1960s, therefore, Lindemann (1969) predicted that the demand for mental health services would increase with the available supply of services and that resources would always fail to meet the needs of the population. The problem could never be resolved by an increase in professional manpower.

The literature of various professional groups in psychiatry assumes that there is a massive level of unmet need for mental health care in the population (Richman and Barry, 1985). Community epidemiological studies have shown that up to 25% of the population may be suffering from a major or minor mental illness – from psychological disturbances, emotional reactions, or demoralization; two out of every five persons suffering from psychosis have never received treatment (Dohrenwend et al. 1980). Kendell (1975), however, questions the assumption made by mental health care professionals that a diagnosis necessitates a plan of clinical action, and defines people as needing medical care. The results of a study by the World Health Organization (1973) showed that it is incorrect to assume that persons with similar symptoms will follow similar courses during their illnesses and have similar outcomes. It tended to confirm Eysenck's (1952) study that many patients with minor psychiatric disorders recover spontaneously without any intervention. The increasing tendency of psychiatric personnel to go beyond their role of treating the mentally ill and to offer advice on a wide range of human issues is, according to Crawford (1980), an example of 'medicalization' of everyday life:

> One aspect of it is an expansion of professional power over a wide range of problems, in particular over deviant behaviours such as drug abuse and

delinquency. Thus, these kinds of problems have been labelled as illness and as symptomatic of psychiatric disorder rather than as a problem of social control. Psychiatry has thus assumed responsibility for problems more properly overseen by legal and religious systems. (Crawford, 1980)

9.5 TWENTIETH CENTURY THEORY AND PRACTICE IN PSYCHIATRIC NURSING

There has been no shortage of theory in 20th century psychiatry. There has, however, been a shortage of people willing or able to put that theory into practice. Theory has often outstripped the established culture of psychiatric nursing, making it impossible to implement it without a radical change in the ethos of care for the mentally ill. Those who practice as psychiatric nurses are the inheritors of a tradition based on custom and practice which determines their role and self-image and which confers on them the security they need to work with the very sick and the incurable. Theorists have failed to recognize how deeply embedded this tradition is and how valued by psychiatric nurses, hence, how unwilling they are to see it undermined. Thinking within psychiatric nursing may be moving rapidly, but theorists gain their security from the advance of ideas; those whom they attempt to influence gain their security from the *status quo* no matter how unsatisfactory.

Psychiatric staff working within a traditional mental hospital may be unable to function separately from it, dependent on, even if oblivious to, the collective coping mechanisms that are deeply entrenched within the institution's structure and culture. There is an in-built resistance to change at both the individual and organizational level. Contradictions within psychiatry are mirrored within psychiatric nursing and nurses have engaged in 'therapeutic practices' based more on the ideological perspective of the nurse than on the needs of the patient (Richman and Barry, 1985). Being innovative in care, measuring effectiveness, basing practice on research, and cost-consciousness are notions that were largely alien to psychiatric nurses in the recent past.

Martin (1984) considers that mental hospitals were and are conservative institutions with a powerful 'hidden culture', essentially maladaptive in the face of change. Within the closed system of the mental hospitals, nurses have neither had nor desired the chance of being exposed to progressive psychiatric ideologies or innovative working practices. They have embodied traditional values of subservience to the system and preservation of the *status quo*. Theirs has been a 'victim role' and by deflecting responsibility for the failures of psychiatry onto doctors, patients, or the institution, have made themselves, some would claim, obstacles to progress (Bowler, 1991).

Georgiades and Phillimore (1975) found that the notion of 'hero-innovators' who could, single-handedly, change the system was a myth. It is merely an evasion to wait for such a person to bring about change within an institution. Milne's (1984) views on the implementation of change were that energy spent on changing practice is wasted if none is expended on rethinking goals and employing dynamic processes which will work to change every aspect of the system. Disjointed attempts at innovation need to be welded into an overall approach to change which is itself innovatory. Responsibility for innovation needs to be corporate rather than invested in 'key individuals'. The training of different professional groups within mental health care in isolation from each other and often from clinical practice has not served patient care well. It has encouraged isolationist thinking and allowed the shifting of responsibility for change from one group to another.

The history of psychiatric nursing suggests that many of those who were appointed to the role of nursing officers to bring about change were, in fact, encouraged and expected to maintain the *status quo* by using cosmetic change strategies only. Subsequent evaluation of services has generated the impression that 'all is well', even though what had been done had been superficial only and the underlying mechanisms and structure remained intact (Prail and Baldwin, 1988).

Men and women coming into mental health nursing at the end of the 20th century represent a very different group of people from those who took up nursing at the beginning or in the middle of the century. They are better educated and more highly skilled; they are also more perceptive, more critical and well able to express their dissatisfactions. In a study of psychiatric nurses working on an admission ward, Handy (1991) found that although their level of commitment was high, the system in which they were working was still such as to produce much disenchantment.

1. Nurses spent most of their time carrying out ward routines such as serving meals and administering medication, while the personal problems that caused patients to be admitted received relatively little attention.
2. The seniority of nursing staff was inversely related to the amount of time they spent with patients and positively related to the amount of time spent on administration or with other disciplines. There was a general tendency for patients to be dealt with by the most inexperienced and the least qualified staff while decisions concerning them were taken by senior staff with less knowledge of them.
3. Patients tended to request oral medication or injections when their symptoms became unbearable in preference to the care provided by nurses.
4. Younger nurses frequently tried to reassure themselves of their usefulness by singling out a few specific patients for special attention. Unfortunately, the wider environment of the psychiatric system often doomed these attempts to failure. When this happened, the nurses often reacted quite defensively and withdrew from patients in order to protect themselves from further disillusionment. Senior staff encour-

aged junior staff to be cynical about the effectiveness of interpersonal skills and paid lip-service to the ideal of individualized care.

5. Nurses felt that little attention had been paid to the problems of implementing the 1982 Syllabus within a hierarchical institutional context dominated by the medical profession and by the treatment techniques of organic psychiatry. Many staff avoid confronting patients' problems because they sense the discrepancy between their public declarations of knowledge and private feelings of inadequacy.

9.6 CARE IN THE COMMUNITY: PITFALLS AND SHORTFALLS

Innovations within mental health care must take into account that there is already a system in existence which has long met the particular ends of many groups of people. In the 19th century, institutionalization of the insane was hailed as a revolution in care, but the reality was that many of the attitudes and practices then current in workhouses, prisons and private institutions were absorbed lock, stock and barrel into the new system. In the 20th century, it would be a mistake to look upon community care as a carte blanche. The question which remains to be answered is how much of the non-therapeutic culture of the mental hospitals will be transferred into community care practice as increasing numbers of institutionally trained staff move away from the hospitals.

The asylums and mental hospitals were accused by their critics of embodying a system of oppressive paternalism; it may be argued that the advocates of the community health care movement were equally paternalistic in their unbending conviction that all clients would prefer to be treated outside hospital settings. Community care became the new Utopia in the 1960s and 1970s. The number of psychiatric hospital beds rapidly decreased and numbers of ex-patients in the community soared. Many of those discharged did not have the necessary social skills to live outside the institutions. 'Liberated' into the community, a liberation which was assumed to be in itself therapeutic, many ex-patients found their lives far grimmer than they had been previously. Communities and families were ill prepared to embrace the deinstitutionalized mentally ill, some of whom simply entered new institutions – prisons, hospitals, boarding houses and half-way houses. Others evaded readmission but were left with no place to live (Gullberg, 1989).

During the 1980s, Government started to ask health carers to encourage their clients to take responsibility for their own health and to be proactive in avoiding ill-health. The NHS was accused of creating a 'dependency culture' so that some people were relying on state agencies to care for them rather than on themselves. Unfortunately, many of the long-term chronically mentally ill are not able to take on board this philosophy of self-help; neither are these clients attractive to staff who now feel that their performance and worth are being evaluated by recovery rates. No professional group is keen to take responsibility for certain categories of mentally ill people, such as the homeless and the long-term mentally ill; the Health Service is being encouraged to transfer as many clients as possible to the Social Services, while both rely increasingly on the independent and voluntary/charitable sectors. While this confusion persists, many mentally ill people end up on the streets or in hostels which do not provide even basic facilities.

In 1979, for every £1 spent by Health and Social Services on mental health, only 12p went on community services and even in 1988, community spending had only increased by 3p to 15p and the rest was still pouring into the hospitals. By the beginning of the 1990s, it was apparent that the transition from hospital to community care had been badly planned and was proving an enormous burden on local resources so that in some parts of the country, large numbers of mentally ill people were not in receipt of any mental health service at all (Social Services Committee, 1990). Sayce (1991) observed that services for the mentally ill were poorly co-ordinated and that some Health Districts were directing funds earmarked for community care in other directions. The quality of residential care provided for some ex-patients amounted to abuse. Sayce cites examples of residents suffering through staff shortages and the imposition of unimaginative regimes. In 14 private homes surveyed in the West Midlands, residents were being offered no social activities at all (West Midlands County Council Economic Development Unit, 1986).

The White Papers 'Caring for People' (1989) and 'Community Care: services for people with a mental handicap and people with a mental illness' (1991) acknowledged that there were anomalies in how community care was being delivered and funded, but reaffirmed that the Government was committed to making community care a reality. 'Caring for People' encouraged the development of locally based services and the collaboration of Health Services, Social Services, and the voluntary and private sectors; the relationship between these different agencies was to be properly co-ordinated to avoid fragmentation of care. The White Paper also stated that short-term hospital admission should remain available for patients for whom there was no realistic alternative.

Getting the structure of community care right is a problem of proportions equalled only by that of ensuring that good practices are adhered to in the community. Traditionally, the system of mental health care in this country has tended to perpetuate the needs of clients, with little effort being made to encourage a functionally independent individual:

> We have used processes which have produced a population of socially incompetent, socially isolated, totally dependent individuals. As a result, tremendous resources are spent today to serve the product of yesterday's services. (Gerhard and Marks, 1980)

Psychiatric services have always tended to be delivered to the 'good patients' who are amenable to psychotherapeutic techniques, boost the morale of staff by their evident progress, and are well suited for the education of students (Levinson, 1969). The result has been a 'heaping up' of services on the most capable clients, to the exclusion of the more severely disordered.

> Nurses along with other mental health care professions have been much more interested in providing services to clients other than the chronically mentally ill. Mental illness represents the only area of practice where the sicker the client is, the worse the quality of treatment. (Moffett, 1988)

Thus the needs of the latter group persist and even grow despite the increasing allocation of resources (Richman and Barry, 1985). Initial findings confirm that it is long-term mentally ill people who are most at risk in the community.

The situation in Britain is mirrored in the USA where the development of community care has given rise to criticism and cynicism akin to reactions in Britain. Vandeburgh (1979) has considered the type of market-economy programme initiated for the care of vulnerable people in the USA as bordering on the unethical:

> The chief beneficiaries of the community psychiatric movement have been psychiatric professionals and nursing home interests. The former group saw in this movement a way to challenge medical psychiatry's virtual monopoly over psychiatric policy, as well as the opportunity for increased influence on its direction. They failed in their first objective, but succeeded in obtaining more lucrative and influential jobs as middle managers and clinicians within the burgeoning psychiatric bureaucracies. And the nursing home industry as a whole has turned a tidy profit from the government transfers, i.e. taxes from the state medical insurance pays for treatment in the community. (Vandeburgh, 1979)

9.7 THE FUTURE FOR MENTAL HEALTH NURSING AND NURSES

9.7.1 The Problems

There are varying and often conflicting opinions about the role and future of mental health nursing as we approach the end of the millenium. Ramon (1991) is not optimistic about the future for psychiatric professionals who, she points out, cannot dissociate themselves from the economic and political climate in which they have to work. She discerns a bleak future ahead:

> It is impossible to escape the sense of a cold welfare climate prevailing throughout the Western World. This has meant cuts in public expenditure and in spending on welfare services. A greater focus on providing services seen to offer good value for money from the point of view of some . . .

is perceived by others as trying to provide a service on the cheap, based on exploitation of a large number of ordinary citizens and attempts to cut down considerably on the responsibility of the collective towards its more vulnerable members. (Ramon, 1991)

Nurses are leaving the institutions in which their profession grew up and had its being for over 150 years at a time when the moral and spiritual climate of the country are quite different from what they were when the asylum system was founded. The Victorian outlook on life was clear-cut and largely untroubled by uncertainty in dealing with the various sections of their society; this has been replaced by an ethos which does not accept that there are universal right answers waiting to be discovered. Instead, each situation has to be considered separately on its own merits before decisions can be taken. In the 19th century, directives from Government were detailed and intended to be implemented nationally without variations; in the late 20th century, social policy has become a 'framework' for action, offering suggestions and outlines to be filled in by local authorities, resulting in a considerable amount of variation.

It is nonetheless true to say that, despite the different societies into which the asylum system and the system of community care were introduced, the motivation for each was not dissimilar. Both initiatives were satisfactory to, if not actually inspired by, the nation's wealth producers. The great manufacturers of the 19th century did not want to be burdened with the costs of outdoor relief for the mentally ill and handicapped; nor at the end of the 20th century did the country's tax-payers and employers wish to shoulder the financial demands of a National Health Service with a boundless capacity to consume monies. The asylum system and community care both represented a step in the dark; they were an experiment backed up by no evidence to suggest that they were likely to prove satisfactory to clients, staff or society. The plans made for the implementation of the two systems were short term only; no consideration was given to long-term objectives or funding. In the case of the asylum system, it was assumed that men and women used to working as farmers, soldiers or servants in the community would easily transfer their labour to the institutions; in the late 20th century, the assumption has been made that staff trained for and accustomed to an institutional context of care will be able to transfer their skills without difficulty into the community setting.

The difference between the asylum system and the system of community care is that the latter is a public venture, whereas the former operated behind closed doors. In the community, nursing practice is on view for all to see and criticize; within the institutions, nurses worked in secrecy and unchallenged. There are many more disciplines caring for patients in the community than there were in the mental hospitals and this creates an atmosphere of competition which is very new to nurses. Public expectations of health professionals become ever greater as do the demands of clients for instant cures. Clients now have rights, know their rights and are prepared to assert them – a very different situation from that of the inmate of a Victorian asylum.

Nurses do not have a strong voice amongst professional groups working with mental health patients because they are disunited. They work in different settings, some in hospitals, some attached to consultants in the community, others to the primary health care team. They belong to a variety of representative bodies such as the RCN, NALGO, COHSE, NUPE, the Psychiatric Nurses' Association and the Community Psychiatric Nurses' Association. They specialize in different areas and have undertaken different training courses. Because of this, mental health nurses are vulnerable and feel more so with the current emphasis on self-help, the rise of the care assistant and the fact that in Europe as a whole, psychiatric nurses constitute only a very small proportion of the health professional work-force, and in some countries do not exist at all. White's (1990) Delphi study suggests that there is uncertainty and pessimism about the future of psychiatric nursing, an uncertainty which may be partly attributed to the fragmentation which is occurring within the profession as it divides into subspecialities.

Project 2000 was eagerly taken up by nurses, but may prove inimical to the interests of mental health nurses. Shared courses are inevitably geared towards the interests and needs of the majority, namely general nurses; what are currently considered to be specialist psychiatric nursing skills may soon be claimed by all nurses. The academic qualifications required for entry into nursing, the 'A'-levels and GCSEs, could be favouring the selection of men and women likely to go into general nursing. In the past, there has always been leeway to select candidates for mental nursing on the grounds of personality and life experience; indeed, a considerable number of entrants have always been mature students against whom the new requirements may discriminate.

The belief that improved practice can be brought about by education alone and by modifying the nursing curriculum has proved mistaken in the past. Merely to include extra subjects such as psychology, sociology, and communication skills in the timetable cannot break the traditional mould of practice. It is unrealistic to expect student nurses, no matter what their capacity to absorb new ideas or their keenness to implement them in the interests of their clients, to be agents of change. Lasting change can only come about as a result of the commitment of all levels of the organization; it has to be encouraged and supported by management which creates the climate in which practitioners can be nurtured through the process of change so that they can nurture their clients.

9.7.2 The Challenges

In an age of competition and professionalization, traditional approaches to health care are being re-evaluated and the pressure on nurses to improve their skills and establish their role in the community is urgent. Clinical Nurse Specialists, appropriately educated with qualifications perhaps to Master's level, must aim to be at the helm of every health care programme, monitoring quality assurance. Their role is to be an educational resource for clients, families and significant others in their clients' lives, providing counselling on issues such as medication, diet, interpersonal relations and individual coping strategies (Pelletier, 1988).

There are evident advantages in the move to train nurses in institutes of higher education. Students are no longer being indoctrinated into the philosophy and practices of just one hospital, but are being given the chance to examine a number of philosophies of care and nursing frameworks. They are being encouraged to establish their own theoretical positions which will best enable them meet the health care needs of their client.

9.7.3 User-Involvement

Much health care provision now centres on the idea of user-involvement which is well established in the USA. The concept behind the catch-phrase is that the consumers of services and those who provide them have abandoned the 'them and us' philosophy upon which the old hospital system was built. It is now accepted that users who have drawn upon health services in the past or who are currently receiving care have a fund of knowledge and useful experience which can be drawn upon to improve the delivery and administration of health services at all levels. User-involvement means that it is both possible and beneficial for consumers and providers to share ideas and work together as equal partners. For some health care professionals, it is an empowering idea with exciting potential for improving services; for others, it is a threat to their idea of themselves and of their role.

9.7.4 Case Management

The White Paper 'Caring for People' (1989) puts forward a model of care widely used in the USA. The case management model is an advanced version of the key-worker system and is only brought into play when the needs of an individual are complex, or significant levels of resources are required for his or her care. It assumes that people from a variety of professional backgrounds will be able to take on the role of Case Manager whose responsibility it is to ensure that the needs of clients are regularly reviewed, that resources are managed efficiently and that the client is assured of prompt referral to an appropriate agency. Treatment thereby becomes a part of the management of care rather than of its delivery; it is planned by a central person who oversees the input of all the professional groups. The Case Manager thus aims to overcome the traditional divisions between health and welfare which have resulted in fragmented and costly delivery of services. Mental health nurses are eminently well-suited to assume the role of Case Manager and need to cultivate the confidence and assertiveness to do so.

9.8 NURSING AND RESEARCH

Despite the considerable attention they have received over the last 150 years, the nature and causes of most mental illnesses are still veiled in mystery. The ongoing uncertainty about how to treat the mentally ill is witnessed by the multiplication of psychiatric practices:

> Today, the most noticeable feature of psychiatric care is the tremendous scope of treatment modalities. The proliferation of forms of treatment – few based upon viable theories or on proven effects – requires the public to accept on the basis of faith that what is being done is useful. (Peplau, 1989)

Research into the effectiveness of any particular form of treatment for chronically mentally sick people faces considerable obstacles:

> Difficulty in identifying treatment goals; difficulty in measuring treatment outcomes; attrition of clients over a relatively short period of time; diversity of psychotherapeutic interventions; and variation among clients with regard to degree of impairment, response to medication, and social support. (Baier, 1988)

The decision to admit a client into hospital or to place him or her on a particular treatment regime is often arbitrary. Selection criteria vary and may include the client's symptoms, economic considerations or the research interests of the consultant or therapist. Under these circumstances, attempting to evaluate the effects of treatment is difficult if not invalid.

Research in nursing is approximately 50 years old and has already provided sufficient well-founded evidence to warrant the conclusion that nursing is a different type of activity from medicine and that nursing interventions have measurable beneficial outcomes. Peplau (1990) sees psychiatric nursing and psychiatry as branches of their respective professions of nursing and medicine; although they have certain features in common, each has separate spheres of responsibility. She finds that nurses:

> Voluntarily assist in the work of psychiatrists; they give medications, monitor reactions, record effects, and recommend adjustments in drug dosages; they discuss cases, share data and plan together so that the patient's total programme makes sense and is as constructive as possible. Nurses know that in addition to human responses, there are physiological and biochemical which can cause anxiety and terror. (Peplau, 1990)

167

She considers that the primary responsibility of nurses is to nurture psychiatric patients in their personal development through the provision of nursing services. To do this, nurses must have an understanding of the range and nature of human responses. Research needs to identify therapeutic interpersonal skills by ascertaining how individual experience mental illness and what support they need in order to have the best quality of life while living with their condition. This includes determining how clients can be helped to live with the side-effects of medication (Babich, 1988).

There is always a danger that research can become part of the 'short termism' which some would consider characteristic of health services management in the 1990s. Funded research projects tend to be of limited duration, 2 or 3 years at most, and once written-up, the researcher may move on to a quite different area of work, leaving the task of implementing his/her findings to others. Where research is undertaken to create an impression of 'scientific' activity when its true purpose is to mask indecision, it becomes a travesty. In common with other disciplines, the aim of most research conducted by mental health nurses is often simply to satisfy the requirements of academic courses. The English National Board would like to incline nurses to see the goal of education and research as improving the quality of patient care, i.e. service-led as opposed to purely academic, and not only the career opportunities of the nurse. Nurses are being asked not to see the writing-up phase as the end of the research process, but as one step in an extended commitment to the subject matter under investigation.

Management, therefore, must now include amongst its aims not only the creation of a climate in which nursing students can learn the skills of nursing care, but also one which will enable research to be carried out in clinical practice and encourage the implementation of research findings. Davis (1990) reviewed a substantial body of research papers written by nurses and about nursing and commented that where nurses had once drawn heavily on the knowledge bases of others, now they are beginning to rely on their own. He concluded that there was sufficient research-based knowledge in place on which to build an applied science able to inform mental health nursing.

9.9 CONCLUSION

Bowler (1991) is optimistic that the 1990s will prove:

A pivotal decade for nursing, one that will bring us more power and a greater recognition within the health care industry. (Bowler, 1991)

Moving patients into the community is an ongoing process, and it may be that some or even many will be moved back again into hospitals or other renamed institutions. The challenge is for mental health nurses to be at the spearhead of the changes which will occur in the Health Services, not lagging behind as has, sadly, been their traditional role. They can no longer afford to follow in the footsteps of other professional groups more assertive than they in defending their interests. Such lack of purpose can only lead to the obliteration of mental health nursing. Should this happen, mental health nurses will probably have nobody to blame but themselves.

Mental health nursing has come a long way since its birth in the asylums of the 19th century. Years of practice and experience have enabled it to develop approaches to the care of mental health patients and acquire wisdom about their management which is of great value and which would be tragic to lose. Despite the many difficulties it has had to confront both in its relationship with the medical profession and because of lack of focus and drive within its own ranks, it has striven in the face of adversity and survived. Nurses are now taking responsibility for their own education, for their own research and for the nature and standards of their own clinical practice. All this represents a huge advance from the first training syllabus for attendants in 1891 – drawn up, taught and examined by doctors, and from the 'Red Handbook' – written by and orientated towards the interests of the medical profession. As the 21st century nears, the aim of mental health nurses must be to transform mental health nursing into the most scientific of the humanities and the most humane of the sciences.

REFERENCES

Babich, K. (1988) Obstacles in research: another point of view. *Journal of Psychosocial Nursing*, **26**, 30–1.

Baier, M. (1988) Why research doesn't yield research. *Journal of Psychosocial Nursing*, **26**, 29–33.

Bowler, J. B. (1991) Transformation into a healthcare environment. *Perspective in Psychiatric Care*, **27**, 34–41.

Crawford, R. (1980) Healthism and the medicalisation of everday life. *International Journal of Health Services*, **10**, 365–88.

Davis, B. D. (1990) Research and psychiatric nursing, in Reynolds W. and Cormack C. *Psychiatric Mental Health Nursing*, eds W. Reynolds and C. Cormack, Chapman & Hall, London, pp. 434–67.

Dohrenwend, B. P., Dohrenwend, B. S., Gould, M. S., Link, B., Neugebauer, R. and Wunsch-Huzig, R. (1980) *Mental Illness in the United States: epidemiological estimates*, Praeger, New York.

Eysenck, H. J. (1952) The effects of psychotherapy: an evaluation. *Journal of Consulting Psychology*, **16**, 319–24.

Georgiades, N. J. and Phillimore, L. (1975) The myth of the hero innovator, in *Behaviour Modification with the Severely Retarded* (eds C. C. Kiernan and F. P. Woodford), Associated Scientific Publishers, London.

Gerhard, R. J. and Marks, A. (1980) Strategies for change: the balanced service system model. *Journal of Pyschiatric Treatment and Evaluation*, **2**, 179–84.

Gullberg, P. L. (1989) A psychiatric nurse's role. *Journal of Psychosocial Nursing*, **27**, 9–13.

Handy, J. (1991) Stress and contradiction in psychiatric nursing. *Human Relations*, **44**, 39–52.

Kendell, R. E. (1975) *The Role of Diagnosis in Psychiatry*, Blackwell Scientific Publications, Oxford.

Levinson, D. J. (1969) Distress in the city – and in the mental health field, in *Distress in the City: esays on the design and administration of urban mental health services* (ed. W. Ryan), The Press of Case Western Reserve University, Cleveland.

Lindemann, E. (1969) Introduction to distress in the city – and inthe mental health-field *Distress in the City: essays on the design and administration of urban mental health services* (ed. W. Ryan), The Press of Case Western Reserve University, Cleveland.

Martin, J. P. (1984) *Hospitals in Trouble*, Basil Blackwell, London.

Milne, D. (1984) Change or innovation in institutions? A constructive role for the 'Realistic Hero Innovator'. *Newsletter*, Division of Clinical Psychology, **43**, 34–7.

Moffett, M. J. (1988) Evolution of psychiatric community care. *Journal of Psycho-social Nursing*, **26**, 17–21.

Pelletier, L. R. (1988) Psychiatric home care. *Journal of Psychosocial Nursing*, **26**, 22–7.

Peplau, H. E. (1989) Future directions in psychiatric nursing from the perspective of history. *Journal of Psychosocial Nursing*, **27**, 18–28.

Peplau, H. E. (1990) Interpersonal relations model: theoretical constructs, principles and general applications, in *Psychiatric Mental Health Nursing*, (eds. W. Reynolds and D. Cormack), Chapman & Hall, London, p. 88.

Prail, T. and Baldwin, S. (1988) Beyond hero-innovation: real change in unreal systems. *Behavioural Psychotherapy*, **16**, 1–14.

Ramon, S. (1991) *Beyond Community Care*, Macmillan in Association with MIND Publications, p. 79.

Richman, A. and Barry, A. (1985) More and more is less and less: the myth of psychiatric need. *British Journal of Psychiatry*, **146**, 164–8.

Sayce, L. (1991) *Waiting for Community Care*, MIND Publications.

Social Services Committee (1990) *Community care: services for people with a mental handicap and people with a mental illness*, Cm. 1522, HMSO, London.

Vandeburgh, H. W. (1979) Critical theory and mental health and illness. Unpublished graduate paper in Sociology, University of California.

West Midlands County Council Economic Development Unit (1986) *The Realities of Home Life*.

White, E. (1990) *The Future of Psychiatric Nursing by the Year 2000: a Delphi study*, Department of Nursing Studies, University of Manchester.

Index